First Aid
 Afloat

Sandra Roberts

First Aid

Afloat

Sandra Roberts

WILEY ✦ NAUTICAL

This edition first published 2011
© 2011 John Wiley & Sons Ltd

Registered office
John Wiley & Sons Ltd, The Atrium, Southern Gate, Chichester, West Sussex, PO19 8SQ, United Kingdom

For details of our global editorial offices, for customer services and for information about how to apply for permission to reuse the copyright material in this book please see our website at www.wiley.com.

Photo credits: page 79: © SHOUT / Alamy; page 108 © Michael J Lewin, Medical Assistant, HMS Illustrious.

Wiley Nautical would like to thank Helly Hansen (**www.hellyhansen.com**) for supplying clothes for the photo shoot.

Library of Congress Cataloging-in-Publication Data
Roberts, Sandra, 1953-
First aid afloat / Sandra Roberts.
p. cm.
Includes index.
ISBN 978-0-470-68207-4 (pbk.)
1. Medicine, Naval. 2. First aid in illness and injury. 3. Medical emergencies. 4. Boats and boating--Health aspects. I. Title.
RC981.R63 2010
616.9'8024--dc22
2010024556

A catalogue record for this book is available from the British Library.

Set in Akzidenz Grotesk
Design by Nigel Pell
Printed in China by Toppan Leefung Printers Ltd

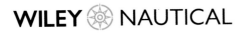

Wiley Nautical – sharing your passion.
At Wiley Nautical we're passionate about anything that happens in, on or around the water. Wiley Nautical used to be called Fernhurst Books and was founded by a national and European sailing champion. Our authors are the leading names in their fields with Olympic gold medals around their necks and thousands of sea miles in their wake. Wiley Nautical is still run by people with a love of sailing, motorboating, surfing, diving, kitesurfing, canal boating and all things aquatic. Visit us online at **www.wileynautical.com** for offers, videos, podcasts and more.

CONTENTS

When out sailing, everyone expects to enjoy the trip without mishaps. Unfortunately, accidents and illness do happen and everyone setting foot on a yacht or small craft should know how to deal with them. Getting help for a casualty takes longer at sea than ashore.

This book presents the fundamental first aid that everyone setting sail should know. It should complement, and not replace, practical instruction. Along with survival, fire and radio training, completing a first aid course should be a part of every yachtsman's basic preparation for sailing. All of these are readily available from a number of organisations.

Read this book and be familiar with its advice before you have to provide first aid to a casualty!

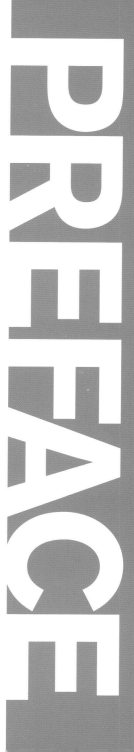

PREFACE

This chapter introduces first aid, with an overview of how to manage an incident occurring at sea that results in injury or illness.

- First Aid

- Anatomy and Physiology

- Managing an Incident

- General Casualty Assessment

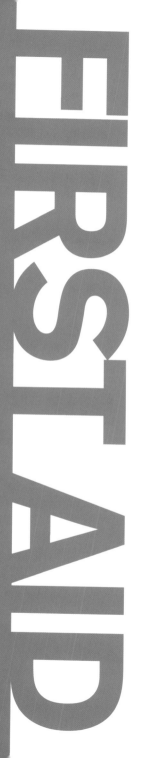

FIRST AID

DEFINITION

First aid is the initial assistance given to a person who has taken ill suddenly or has been injured in an accident.

AIMS AND OBJECTIVES

The aims and objectives of first aid may be summarised as **preserving** life, **preventing** further harm and **promoting** recovery.

PRIORITIES

In any first aid situation, the priority in terms of the casualty is always to ensure they have a clear airway and are able to breathe. However, the rescuer first needs to make sure the environment is safe.

ANATOMY AND PHYSIOLOGY

Having a basic understanding of how the body works will enable the first aider to understand what is happening to the casualty and why the actions they take actually assist the casualty.

Oxygen is required by all the cells in the body. Without it, we die. In first aid, efforts are made to ensure oxygen continues to reach vital organs.

Oxygen is breathed in, and is then circulated around the body in the blood by the pumping action of the heart. If breathing or circulation is affected by illness or injury, this will result in body tissue being deprived of oxygen and it will be permanently damaged or even die. Brain cells start to die off after a few minutes. Without oxygen, the heart stops working.

Blood vessels that carry the oxygenated blood to the tissues are called arteries. When an **artery** is cut the blood spurts out with each heartbeat and, because it contains oxygen, it is bright red. Blood vessels that take blood back to the heart are called **veins**. When these are cut the blood is not under such great pressure and does not contain oxygen, so it is a darker red and does not spurt, but flows or gushes out. **Capillaries** are the smallest blood vessels and when they are damaged they ooze blood.

When a casualty is bleeding it is important to recognise which type of bleeding is happening, as this will dictate the speed of action taken.

The musculoskeletal system is made up of bones, muscles, tendons and ligaments. The skeleton provides a framework to support and move the body and also gives some protection to internal structures. Muscles move the skeleton and are attached to bones by tendons. Ligaments bind bone ends together in joints and also support internal organs.

A first aider does not need to know the individual names of these different structures. When describing an injury it is best to use simple terminology such as "thigh" or "upper arm".

MANAGING AN INCIDENT

At any first aid incident, the rescuer will follow a plan of action. This will take place in any setting, either afloat or ashore. The situation and casualty will be assessed, help sought, the casualty treated and any aftermath dealt with. The time it takes, and the methods used, may change according to the circumstances and the severity of the situation, but this process will always be carried out.

Assessing the situation	Check that there is no danger to self or the casualty, and if there is, make it safe. Remember that the danger may not be obvious. Think hygiene and personal safety. Think about the immediate space around your casualty (e.g. spillages on deck, trip hazards, broken glass, wood splinters). Think about the dangers peculiar to your own environment (e.g. swinging boom, open hatches, loose ropes, rough seas). Look for clues to work out what has happened.

Assessing the casualty

The initial assessment of your casualty is called the primary survey. This is the priority in any first aid situation.

Does the casualty have an **airway**? Is the casualty **breathing**? Remember that if the casualty is able to speak or make sounds, they are breathing.

What injuries are there? Can you see any obvious bleeding or broken bones? What can the casualty tell you?

Getting help

Shout for help so others on board are alerted.

Ensure everyone on board knows how to summon help on the radio in an emergency.

When calling for help, the information required will be the identity of the yacht and your location, what has happened and what help is required, how many casualties there may be and what their injuries are.

Treating the casualty

Constantly be aware of any danger to you and your casualty while treating them.

Remember: the priorities of first aid are AIRWAY and BREATHING.

This book shows how to recognise and carry out basic treatments for a number of injuries and illnesses.

Dealing with the aftermath

This includes the completion of reports in log books, restocking first aid kits, and cleaning up body fluid spillages in a safe manner.

As well as dealing with practical issues, consideration needs to be given to emotional needs. If a major incident has been dealt with, this can be very traumatic for all involved. Though you may react well and deal with the situation at the time, afterwards it is important not to be afraid to talk about how you feel.

GENERAL CASUALTY ASSESSMENT

After assessing and treating any obvious injuries a casualty may have, it is important to check them over physically in case they have sustained other injuries.

THE SECONDARY SURVEY

The secondary survey establishes what other injuries the casualty may have that were not identified initially. The casualty may be able to tell you but you may have to search for them. The secondary survey is also called the "top to toe" or "head to toe" survey because it describes what the first aider does.

The first aider should work down the body from the head, feeling for lumps and bumps and looking for wounds. Note if it is tender to touch anywhere. Ideally, this should be done wearing gloves to protect the rescuer from contact with blood or other body fluids.

As well as looking for other injuries, the survey may help to establish the reason why someone has become ill or is unconscious. The first aider becomes a detective. Items found in the casualty's pockets or smells on the casualty's breath may help identify the problem.

If a casualty is unconscious they should be placed in the recovery position before the secondary survey is carried out.

GENERAL CASUALTY ASSESSMENT
(continued)

OBSERVATIONS

While waiting for help to arrive, you will need to monitor the condition of the casualty. You may need to write down what you find, or get someone else to do it for you. The frequency will depend on the condition of the casualty but usually most observations will be done every ten minutes. Breathing checks will be more frequent than this. Your checks will include the following.

Breathing	Is the casualty actually breathing? Check this every one to two minutes in a casualty who is unconscious. How fast is the breathing? Count the breaths per minute. Is it deep or shallow breathing? Is the breathing noisy? Is the casualty coughing? Is the chest moving evenly? Is the casualty distressed when breathing?
Level of consciousness	Use the letters **AVPU** to remember what needs to be done. A – is the casualty **alert**? Can they tell you their name and where they are? V – does the casualty respond to your **voice** when you ask them to do something? How well do they respond? P – does the casualty respond to simple **physical stimulation** like shoulder shaking? If not, do they respond to pain? U – is the casualty **unresponsive**?

Pupils	In the eyes, are the casualty's pupils the same size and shape? Do the pupils react by constricting quickly when a light is shone into them? Is the reaction the same in both eyes?
Pulse	The pulse may be felt at the side of the wrist near the base of the thumb. In a seriously ill, very cold or injured casualty, feel at the neck at the side of the voice box. What is the pulse count per minute? Is it regular? Is it strong or weak?
Skin	What colour is the casualty's skin? Is it pale and ashen, or red and flushed? Is there any blueness around the mouth and face? Is the skin hot or cold to touch? Dry or wet? Are any marks visible?
Wounds and fractures	Is the wound still bleeding? Check the circulation below the dressing or fracture. If the skin is pressed, does it go white then come back to pink quickly on release of pressure? Does the limb feel cold to touch? Is the casualty complaining of pins and needles?

This is all important information about the casualty that you will need to pass on when medical help is sought. This is in addition to all the other information you will be required to give regarding the casualty's injuries and the first aid that has been carried out already.

This chapter details how to manage life threatening situations, some of which may require resuscitation.

- Basic Life Support

- Drowning

- The Choking Casualty

- The Unconscious Casualty

- Shock

RESUSCITATION

BASIC LIFE SUPPORT

Heart disease is the main cause of death in the United Kingdom. It may be slow and progressive, often with no external signs or symptoms until illness suddenly presents.

A heart attack is a major cause of a cardiac arrest, which is when the heart has stopped beating and blood and oxygen stop circulating around the body. When the heart has stopped beating, the casualty will also not be breathing.

These functions are taken over by the rescuer in an attempt to keep oxygen supplied to vital organs, in particular the brain and the heart itself. This is known as cardiopulmonary resuscitation (CPR). Where no equipment is used to do this, it is also known as basic life support (BLS).

It is important that the rescuer commences BLS immediately. Over time, the techniques used to do this have been simplified to make it easier for the rescuer. The sequence of events can be remembered by using **DR ABC**.

D is for danger – is it safe for the casualty, the rescuer and bystanders?

R is for response – does the casualty respond?

A is for airway – is the airway open, allowing the casualty to breathe?

B is for breathing – is the casualty breathing on their own?

C is for circulation – is the heart pumping blood around the body?

RESPONSE

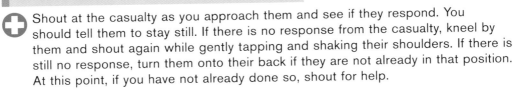
Shout at the casualty as you approach them and see if they respond. You should tell them to stay still. If there is no response from the casualty, kneel by them and shout again while gently tapping and shaking their shoulders. If there is still no response, turn them onto their back if they are not already in that position. At this point, if you have not already done so, shout for help.

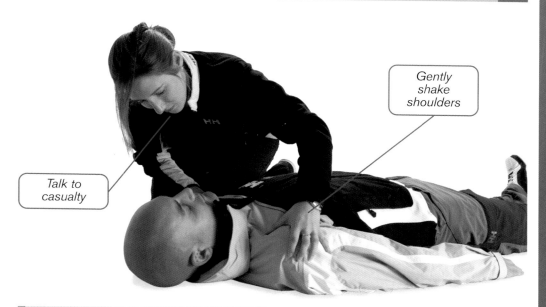

Gently
shake
shoulders

Talk to
casualty

AIRWAY

➕ Make sure the casualty has an open
airway. Place your hand on their
forehead and gently tilt the head
back. Place your fingertips under
the chin and lift the chin up.
This action opens the
airway by moving
the tongue away
from the airway
entrance.

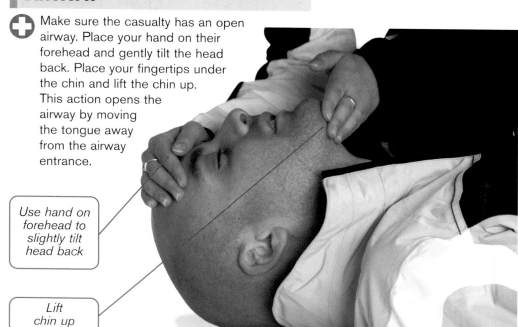

Use hand on
forehead to
slightly tilt
head back

Lift
chin up

19

BREATHING CHECK

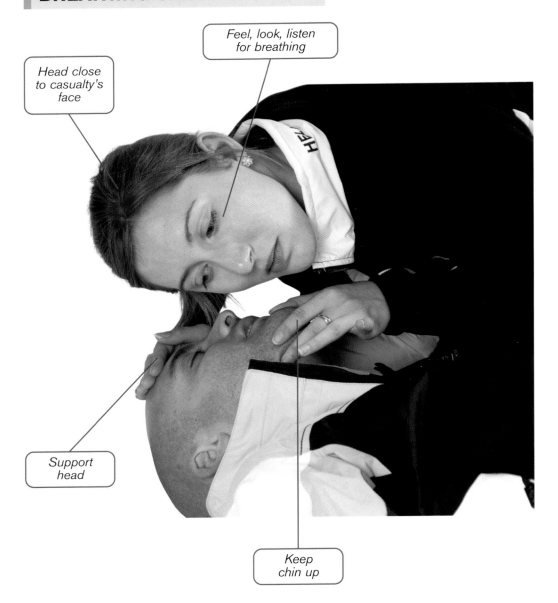

Feel, look, listen for breathing

Head close to casualty's face

Support head

Keep chin up

Now check for breathing. With your head next to the casualty's face, keep the chin supported and look, listen and feel for evidence of normal breathing for no longer than ten seconds. Can you feel breath on your cheek? Can you see the chest rise and fall? Can you hear any sounds?

Do not confuse irregular noisy gasps for normal breathing. If you doubt that breathing is normal, act as if it is not and continue with resuscitation.

If the casualty is not breathing, raise the alarm at once if you have not already done so. This may mean leaving the casualty to do so.

COMPRESSIONS

It's now time to start chest compressions to restore circulation and make sure the casualty's brain continues to receive oxygen while you wait for help. Kneeling by the side of the casualty, place the heel of one hand in the centre of their chest. Place the heel of the other hand on top of the heel of the first. Interlock your fingers and raise them off the chest, ensuring no pressure is applied on the ribs. No pressure should be put on the lower end of the breastbone or the upper abdomen.

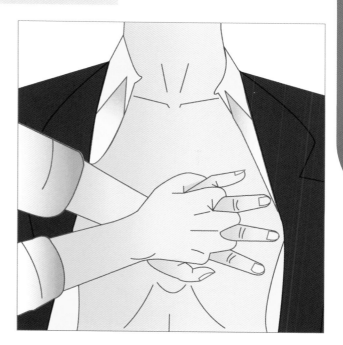

➕ Positioned vertically over the casualty, with your arms locked straight and your hand, elbow and shoulder in line, press down on the breastbone to a depth of 4-5cm. After each compression release all the pressure on the chest, letting it return to its original position, but do not remove your hands from the chest.

➕ Repeat this at a rate of 100 per minute. Compression and release should take an equal amount of time. Complete 30 compressions.

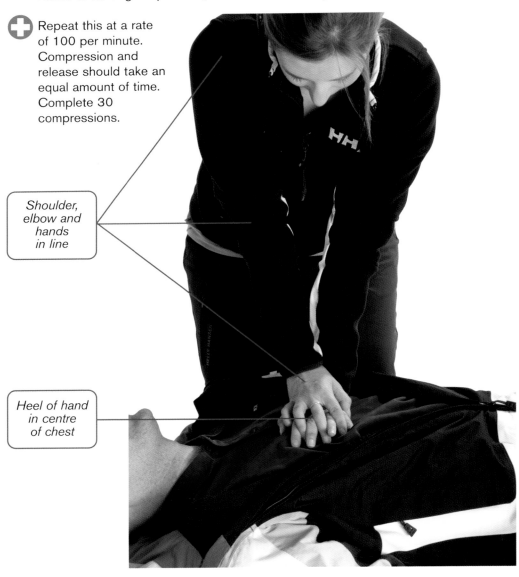

Shoulder, elbow and hands in line

Heel of hand in centre of chest

RESCUE BREATHS

➕ After 30 compressions, open the casualty's airway using the "head tilt, chin lift" method. Pinch the soft part of the nose using the thumb and index finger of one hand. Maintain the chin lift with the other hand, keeping the casualty's mouth open. Take a normal breath and place your lips around the casualty's mouth, making sure there is a good seal. Blow steadily into the mouth and watch for the chest to rise as in normal breathing. This takes about one second. Take your mouth away and watch for the chest to fall as the air comes out. Repeat this once more. This completes two effective rescue breaths.

➕ If rescue breaths did not make the chest rise and fall, before you make the next attempt at breaths, check the casualty's mouth for visible obstructions and ensure that the head tilt and chin lift are adequate. Do not attempt more than two breaths before returning to compressions.

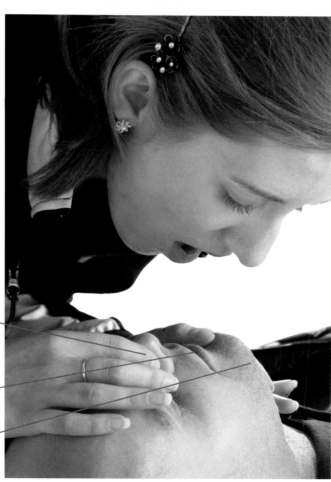

Pinch nostrils to close

Open mouth

Support chin

BASIC LIFE SUPPORT *(continued)*

➕ Return to the chest without delay and give 30 more compressions. Continue using a ratio of 30 compressions to two breaths.

➕ Do not interrupt the resuscitation. It is extremely unlikely that the casualty will recover with CPR alone. Only stop CPR if you are in danger or exhausted, or help arrives to take over from you.

➕ The rescuer will become tired after only a minute of CPR. Where two rescuers are present they should take turns, swapping over every two minutes, attempting to do so without any break in the CPR.

➕ If you are unable to do ventilations because of a risk of infection, the presence of blood or vomit, suspicion of poisoning or because you just choose not to, it is important still to do compressions. Continue compressions without any break until help arrives.

➕ The casualty needs to be on a hard surface so may need to be moved from a bunk onto the deck.

DROWNING

➕ In drowning incidents, after discovering the casualty is not breathing, basic life support should be commenced.

➕ The sequence of events is slightly modified, however. Unlike in a sudden collapse from cardiac arrest, a casualty who has been rescued from drowning has not been breathing and does not have oxygen in their blood to be circulated. This lack of oxygen is what causes the heart to stop.

➕ If you are alone with the casualty, give them five rescue breaths and then continue with compressions and ventilations at a ratio of 30 compressions to two ventilations for one minute, before leaving the casualty and raising the alarm. Where another rescuer is available to raise the alarm, give five rescue breaths and continue with compressions and breaths at a ratio of 30:2 until help arrives.

A SUMMARY OF ADULT BASIC LIFE SUPPORT

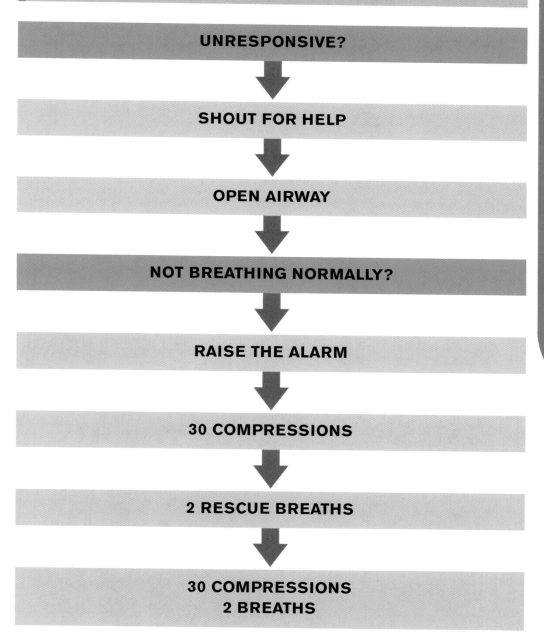

UNRESPONSIVE?

SHOUT FOR HELP

OPEN AIRWAY

NOT BREATHING NORMALLY?

RAISE THE ALARM

30 COMPRESSIONS

2 RESCUE BREATHS

**30 COMPRESSIONS
2 BREATHS**

THE CHOKING CASUALTY

CAUSE

Choking occurs when a foreign object enters the airway and causes a partial or complete blockage.

THREAT

When the airway is completely blocked, the casualty is unable to breathe or make any sound. Blockages usually occur when the person is breathing in, and this leaves little air in the lungs for the casualty to expel, to remove the object themselves.

RECOGNITION

It is important not to confuse this with other emergencies where the casualty appears to have difficulty breathing. If the obstruction is mild, the casualty will be able to answer or cough and will recover without assistance. If the casualty is unable to answer they may clutch or point to their throat to indicate the problem.

Choking frequently occurs during eating.

RESPONSE

The role of the rescuer is to attempt to dislodge the blockage by forcing residual air out from the lungs.

➕ If the casualty is still conscious, attempt to dislodge the object. Stand beside the casualty and lean them forward, supporting them with an arm. Give up to five sharp blows between the shoulder blades with the heel of your other hand.

Check after each slap to see if the object has dislodged.

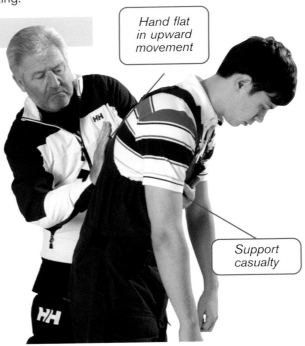

Hand flat in upward movement

Support casualty

➕ If this does not relieve the situation, the next technique to try is the abdominal thrust. Stand behind the casualty and lean them forward, putting both arms around the upper part of their abdomen. Clench a fist and place it midway between the belly button and the bottom end of the breastbone. Grasp this hand with the other and pull sharply upwards and inwards. Repeat up to five times, checking after each thrust to see if the object has dislodged.

➕ If the obstruction is not relieved, continue alternating five abdominal thrusts with five back slaps.

➕ If the casualty becomes unconscious, commence CPR.

Hands placed midway between ribs and navel

Thumb tucked in

Grip with hand

THE CHOKING CASUALTY *(continued)*

AFTERCARE

Abdominal thrusts may cause serious internal injury. Medical advice should be sought if they have been carried out, and the casualty should be observed for evidence of internal injury.

Following successful treatment for choking, foreign material may remain in the upper or lower respiratory tract and cause complications later. If the casualty has a persistent cough, difficulty swallowing or the sensation of an object still being stuck in their throat, they should always seek medical attention.

THE UNCONSCIOUS CASUALTY

CAUSE

There are numerous possible causes for someone being unconscious. These may be related to injury or trauma, drugs, alcohol or other poisoning, medical conditions or environmental conditions.

THREAT

The immediate threat to life in an unconscious casualty comes from the tongue falling back and obstructing the airway, thus preventing breathing, and from the inhalation of vomit.

RESPONSE

The role of the rescuer is to position the casualty to secure their airway, and to assess the possible causes of the unconsciousness.

Follow the **DR ABC** routine and check that the casualty is actually unconscious. Even if they respond but are very drowsy, continue with the recovery position. If there is no response, open the airway and check that breathing is present. Once breathing is confirmed, the casualty must be placed in a safe position to ensure the airway remains open to allow breathing, and to help prevent the inhalation of vomit.

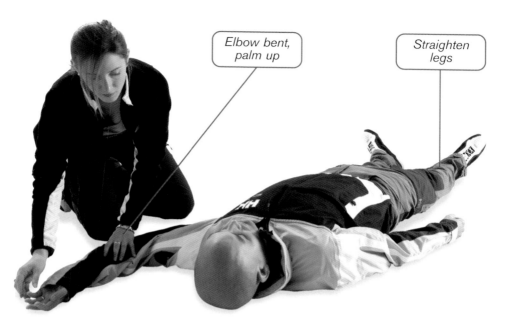

Elbow bent, palm up

Straighten legs

➕ Kneel next to the casualty and straighten both their legs. Remove their spectacles if they are wearing them. Quickly check there is nothing in the casualty's pockets that may cause them harm when they are turned onto their side. Place the arm closest to you out at right angles to the body with the elbow bent and the palm uppermost.

➕ Bring the casualty's opposite arm across their chest and hold the back of their hand against their cheek with your own palm. Do not let go. This hand supports the head as the casualty is turned.

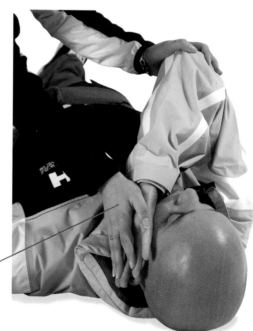

Support hand against cheek

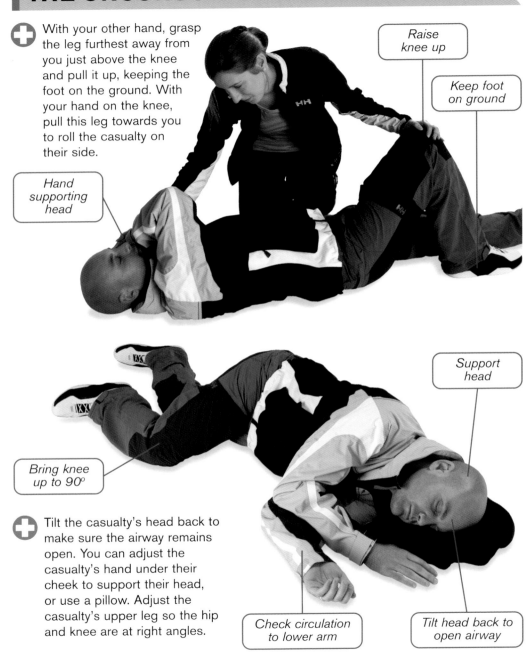

➕ With your other hand, grasp the leg furthest away from you just above the knee and pull it up, keeping the foot on the ground. With your hand on the knee, pull this leg towards you to roll the casualty on their side.

Raise knee up

Keep foot on ground

Hand supporting head

Support head

Bring knee up to 90°

➕ Tilt the casualty's head back to make sure the airway remains open. You can adjust the casualty's hand under their cheek to support their head, or use a pillow. Adjust the casualty's upper leg so the hip and knee are at right angles.

Check circulation to lower arm

Tilt head back to open airway

AFTERCARE

The casualty's breathing must be checked frequently – every one to two minutes. If they are not breathing, roll them onto their back and commence resuscitation.

If the casualty has to be kept in the recovery position for more than 30 minutes, turn them onto the opposite side to relieve pressure on the lower arm.

Any injury the casualty has suffered may determine which side they should be laid on in the recovery position but securing the airway always takes priority over any injury. There is more detail on this in *Chapter 4: Injuries.*

Never leave an unconscious casualty alone unless it is necessary in order to raise the alarm. Cover them to prevent heat loss and protect them from the environment as needed.

Do not move the casualty unless they are in danger as this may cause further harm.

Assess the casualty for signs of injury or possible cause of the unconsciousness, and monitor their pulse. These aftercare observations are detailed in the General Casualty Assessment section in chapter 1.

SHOCK

Shock is a lessening of the vital activities of the body. It is a physical condition and should not be confused with emotional shock.

It may result in unconsciousness and death if not managed immediately. The speed of onset of shock varies and may not depend on the severity of the injury.

CAUSE

Shock has many different causes. It may be the result of severe pain, injury, allergy, infection, fluid loss, or medical conditions such as heart attack.

Fluid loss may be from bleeding, diarrhoea and vomiting, or burns.

SHOCK *(continued)*

RECOGNITION

There are many different **signs and symptoms of shock**, and it is important to be aware of these when dealing with a casualty. In the early stages of an emergency these signs are easily missed.

They may include **drowsiness, confusion, agitation and dizziness**. These are due to a lack of oxygen reaching the brain. **Pale, cold, clammy skin** occurs as the body withdraws the blood supply from the skin and diverts it to vital organs. **Thirst, nausea and vomiting, rapid shallow breathing and a fast weak pulse** can also be found in a shocked casualty.

RESPONSE

Always remember to check the airway is open and that the casualty is breathing.

1 Lay the casualty down flat on their back and **raise their legs** if the injury allows this. This helps blood flow to the core body organs.

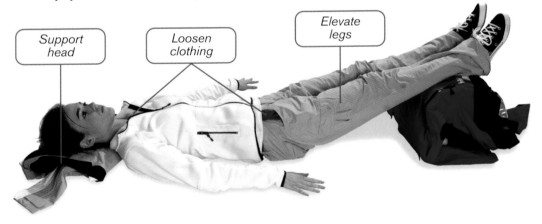

Support head

Loosen clothing

Elevate legs

2 **Do not move** the casualty unless they are in danger as this may worsen the shock, but if they are outside, **protect them from the elements**. Cover the casualty to **prevent them losing heat** but do not over warm them. If possible, lie them on something rather than directly onto a cold deck. Constantly reassure the casualty and try to keep them comfortable.

Loosen tight clothing at the neck and waist to aid breathing. Moisten the casualty's lips but do not allow them to eat or drink. This is likely to cause vomiting and the airway may become compromised.

Remember that shock can happen at any time during an emergency. It's important to keep monitoring the casualty even if their condition appears to stabilise.

This chapter details
bleeding and burns, and
outlines how to recognise
the different types and the
first aid they require.

- External Bleeding

- Internal Bleeding

- Nose Bleeds

- Burns (Hot and Cold)

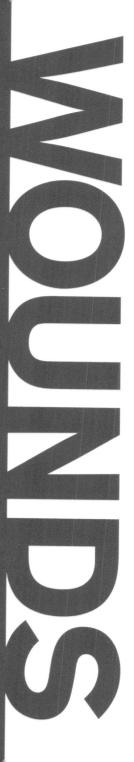

EXTERNAL BLEEDING

RECOGNITION

Bleeding may be minor or life threatening. It is important to be able to recognise different types of bleeding in order to determine the severity, and the speed of response required. The appearance of the blood will vary depending on whether the blood is going to or from the heart.

Arterial blood is being pumped from the heart and contains oxygen. It is bright red and spurting. It is life threatening and requires urgent action.

Venous blood is on its way back to the heart, having delivered oxygen to the body. It is dark red, and flows, gushes or pools. Although rapid action is needed, venous bleeding is not as urgent as arterial bleeding.

Capillary blood, which is from the smallest of the blood vessels, oozes out. This is minor bleeding, for example from a graze.

RESPONSE

At sea, where medical help is not readily available, it is vital that all seafarers know how to stop bleeding that is potentially life threatening. To control external bleeding, two things are needed – **PRESSURE** and **ELEVATION**.

➕ Where bleeding is visible, the type of bleeding and the exact location of the wound needs to be identified. Check whether there are any penetrating objects. If there are, do not remove them as this could worsen the situation.

➕ Remember: a first aid kit is not required to control bleeding. It is pressure and elevation that control bleeding.

➕ Apply a dressing directly over the wound. It does not matter if the dressing looks bulky or unsightly. The intention is to stop the bleeding, and a neatly secured dressing pad and bandage will not do this. Any pad may be used if first aid dressings are not immediately to hand.

➕ Continue to apply pressure directly on the wound even when the dressing has been secured, as the dressing by itself will not stop severe bleeding. Do not remove any dressings applied. If blood soaks through, add another dressing on top, up to a maximum of two.

➕ Where there is a penetrating object, padding should be applied at the base of the object and held in place. No pressure must be put on the object, and no attempt made to remove it.

➕ Apply direct pressure to the wound. This needs to be firm and constant. If possible, get the casualty to apply initial pressure themselves, while you protect yourself from blood contact. This may be done by putting on gloves or just using a barrier that prevents direct contact with the bleeding wound.

➕ If a foreign object is present, pressure should be applied to the wound at the base of the penetrating object. Try to elevate the wound as high above the level of the heart as possible. This helps to slow the flow of blood and allow clotting to take place. With limbs, this is easy.

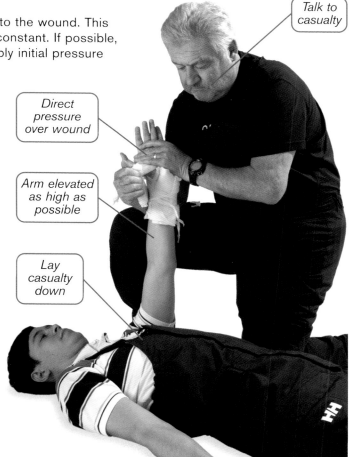

Talk to casualty

Direct pressure over wound

Arm elevated as high as possible

Lay casualty down

➕ In an arterial bleed, direct pressure to the wound may not be sufficient to stop the bleeding. If the dressings applied are soaked in blood, and direct pressure does not appear to stop the bleeding, the flow of blood must be controlled by restricting it at a point distant to the wound. This is called a pressure point and is where an artery is lying close enough to the surface to be felt, but can be compressed against an adjacent bone. This compression will restrict the blood flow through it.

✚ If bleeding is in the leg, there is a pressure point in the groin (**femoral artery**).
If it is in the arm, there is a pressure point in the upper arm (**brachial artery**).

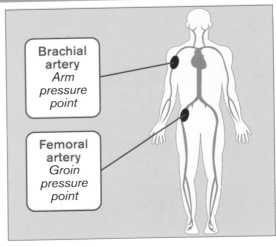

Brachial artery
Arm pressure point

Femoral artery
Groin pressure point

✚ It is important that elevation is still used while indirect pressure is being applied. Direct pressure should also be maintained while indirect pressure is being carried out. A single first aider is able to do this if the bleed is in the arm but, for a leg bleed, the first aider will need assistance to maintain both direct and indirect pressure. If alone, they should maintain the indirect pressure. Indirect pressure must only be maintained for a maximum of ten minutes, because blood supply is being cut off from the whole limb, not just the wound, and tissue is being deprived of oxygen.

✚ If pressure is maintained for longer than ten minutes, healthy tissue will start to die and the limb will be put at risk. At the end of ten minutes, very slowly release the indirect pressure, all the time maintaining pressure over the wound itself, together with elevation. Indirect pressure may be reapplied for a further ten minutes once the colour of the limb has returned to normal.

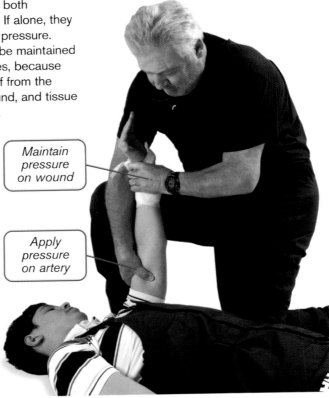

Maintain pressure on wound

Apply pressure on artery

➕ Make sure the casualty is in a safe position. Sitting on the deck is safest but shock will happen quickly if the bleed is severe, so the casualty should be laid in the shock position. Remember that the casualty will be unable to maintain adequate pressure and elevation for long on their own, as they become weaker and more shocked.

➕ If the casualty becomes unconscious, place them in the recovery position while continuing to stop the bleeding. Try to keep the wound elevated as high as possible. For example, if the wound is on the left arm, the unconscious casualty should be placed on their right side. This will allow the arm to be raised as high as possible, as well as allowing easy access to the upper arm if indirect pressure is needed.

Injury uppermost to continue elevation

Maintain direct and artery pressure

➕ When bleeding cannot be controlled by direct or indirect pressure, and blood loss has become life threatening, only then should a tourniquet be used. A tourniquet is a tight, encircling dressing that completely restricts all blood flow to a limb. It should be placed as close to the wound as possible to limit tissue loss and be tied as tightly as possible. Once in place, it stays there and should not be released. Radio medical advice should always be sought if a tourniquet is used or being considered for use. Make a record of the time the tourniquet was applied.

Airway open

Recovery position

➕ Keeping the casualty still will help to slow down blood flow so, unless they are in danger, the casualty should not be moved until the bleeding is under control. If the bleed has been from an arm wound, the arm can be immobilised using a sling to keep it still or maintain elevation.

QUICK GUIDE TO EXTERNAL BLEEDING CONTROL

Casualty safety	Sit or lie the casualty down. Place them directly in the shock position if the bleed is major.
Identify the type of bleeding	To determine the urgency and seriousness of the situation. Arterial? Venous?
Identify the wound	To ensure direct pressure is placed in the correct place.
Identify penetrating objects	To ensure pressure is placed at the base of the object and not on top of it.
Apply direct pressure	Must be placed directly over the bleeding wound to restrict blood flow and encourage blood clotting.
Elevate the wound	Restricts blood flow, reduces blood loss and allows clotting to take place at the wound.
Apply indirect pressure	To restrict the blood flow when it is not possible to control bleeding by direct pressure. Maximum time to hold is ten minutes. Release slowly. May be reapplied.
Apply tourniquet	A last resort in life threatening bleeding only. Goes on and stays on. Place as close to the wound as possible.
Monitor injury	Check the circulation beyond the wound and bandaging. If necessary, release pressure slightly from an encircling dressing. Check for renewed bleeding.
Monitor casualty	Check for shock and manage immediately if recognised. Check pulse and breathing.

The dressings should be checked for evidence of renewed bleeding. The circulation to the limb below the wound should be monitored. If the limb below the dressing is cold to touch, or looks pale or blue, and the casualty complains of numbness or tingling, the circulation could be restricted. It may have been damaged by the injury or be restricted by a dressing that is too tight. It may be necessary to release the pressure on an encircling dressing if it is too tight.

INTERNAL BLEEDING

CAUSE

Injury or illness may result in internal bleeding.

RECOGNITION

If blood cannot escape from the body, internal bleeding can only be recognised by the symptoms of shock that the casualty will be displaying. The casualty may also be in pain.

In some situations evidence of internal bleeding may be seen, for example coughing up blood after a chest injury or passing blood in urine after a back injury. The blood is escaping from the body through an orifice, or opening. The appearance of the blood will depend on the cause of the bleeding and its location.

A history of injury or illness may also lead to suspicion of internal bleeding. For example, an injury to the chest or abdomen may appear to result only in bruising and tenderness. The casualty should be monitored, however, in case internal injury has occurred, resulting in bleeding.

RESPONSE

The first aider should manage any shock and monitor the casualty. It is vital to seek radio medical advice.

NOSE BLEEDS

CAUSE

Nose bleeds usually happen as a result of trauma. They may also occur when blood vessels in the nose burst as a result of over enthusiastic nose blowing and picking, infection and high blood pressure.

RESPONSE

Most nose bleeds can be controlled by simple measures.

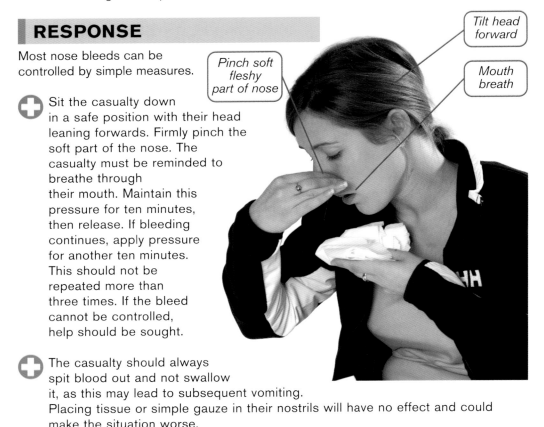

Pinch soft fleshy part of nose

Tilt head forward

Mouth breath

➕ Sit the casualty down in a safe position with their head leaning forwards. Firmly pinch the soft part of the nose. The casualty must be reminded to breathe through their mouth. Maintain this pressure for ten minutes, then release. If bleeding continues, apply pressure for another ten minutes. This should not be repeated more than three times. If the bleed cannot be controlled, help should be sought.

➕ The casualty should always spit blood out and not swallow it, as this may lead to subsequent vomiting. Placing tissue or simple gauze in their nostrils will have no effect and could make the situation worse.

➕ Once the bleeding has stopped, do not allow the casualty to blow their nose, pick at blood clots in the nostril or sniff hard, as this may restart the bleed.

➕ If the casualty becomes shocked they should be placed in the shock position, but with their head and shoulders raised.

BURNS

DEFINITION

A burn is tissue damage caused by heat or cold.

HEAT BURNS

CAUSE OF

Dry heat, wet heat, electricity, chemicals, friction and radiation may all result in heat burns.

RECOGNITION

Burns may be described in a number of ways. The **severity** of a burn depends on both its **depth** and its **area**.

The depth of a burn may be **superficial**, where the skin is red and tender. A **partial** thickness burn is red and tender but also has blistering. The appearance of a **deep** burn will depend on its cause. It may appear white, or black and charred. The nerves are damaged and the casualty may not have any sensation in the burn.

The area of the body affected by a burn can be estimated by using the size of the casualty's palm as a template; this represents approximately one per cent of the body's surface area.

Burns may also be defined as **complex** because of the part of the body affected. These include burns to the face, neck and joints, particularly the hands. Burns in the genital and anal areas are considered complex because of the increased risk of infection.

This hand shows superficial burns as well as partial thickness burns, where the blisters have been burst during wound cleaning and assessment in a hospital.

Blisters should never be burst by the first aider.

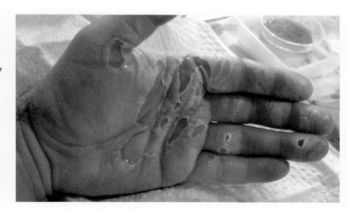

RESPONSE

Remove the casualty from the source of the heat. The burn should be **cooled** for a minimum of ten minutes. It is preferable to do this under running water to carry the heat away. If a burn is soaked in a bowl of water, the water should be replaced periodically, as the burn will actually heat up the water. Never put ice in cooling water or use an ice pack on a burn as this causes further tissue damage. If the burn has been caused by a chemical, it should always be washed off the skin and never soaked in water as this will still contain the chemical.

Remove restrictions like rings, watches and other jewellery, as swelling will occur very quickly. Clothing that may be charred and burnt into the skin should not be pulled off, as this will further damage the tissue. If hot water has been spilt onto clothing and it is not stuck to the skin, you should remove the clothing as contact with the hot wet material will continue to burn. Burns to the mouth may be cooled by rinsing with cold water, ensuring it is spat out and not swallowed.

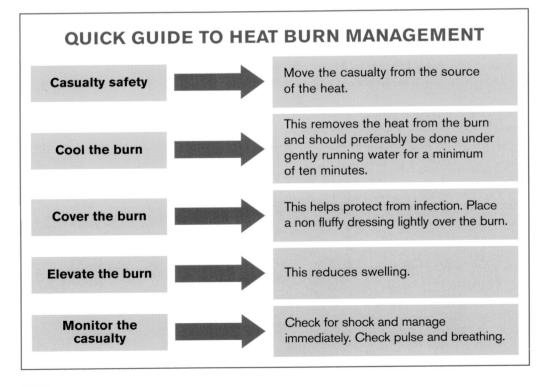

QUICK GUIDE TO HEAT BURN MANAGEMENT

Casualty safety	Move the casualty from the source of the heat.
Cool the burn	This removes the heat from the burn and should preferably be done under gently running water for a minimum of ten minutes.
Cover the burn	This helps protect from infection. Place a non fluffy dressing lightly over the burn.
Elevate the burn	This reduces swelling.
Monitor the casualty	Check for shock and manage immediately. Check pulse and breathing.

Once cooled, the burn should be **covered** lightly with a non fluffy dressing. A triangular bandage from a first aid kit is useful for this. You can also use clingfilm from the galley or any clean, non fluffy fabric such as a clean tea towel. Burnt hands and feet may be placed inside an unused plastic food bag. Where possible, elevate the burn to help reduce swelling.

A minor burn can then be treated using a burn cream from the first aid kit. If the burn is severe enough to warrant getting further advice, however, you should never use burn cream. If you do, it will disguise the burn and will need to be cleaned off before the burn can be fully assessed. This will cause unnecessary pain for the casualty.

COLD BURNS

CAUSE OF

Contact with ice, chemicals or cold environmental conditions may result in cold burns. Frostbite is detailed in the chapter on environmental conditions *(pages 78-79)*.

RECOGNITION

Initially the skin is pale, but the colour may progress to blackened. The casualty may complain of numbness or pins and needles but not have pain. The skin feels cold and hard to the touch.

RESPONSE

Remove all restricting jewellery, watches etc. The treatment is then to **slowly rewarm** the cold tissue. This is done by immersion in warm water, keeping the temperature constant at 40°C. The cold tissue should never be rubbed to warm it, as this can further damage tissue.

There will be pain when the tissue warms up, and the casualty may need a strong painkiller.

As with a hot burn, the tissue may swell, so when possible it should be elevated. It should also be covered by a light, non stick dressing.

QUICK GUIDE TO COLD BURN MANAGEMENT

Rewarm the burn	→	This should be done slowly and gently.
Put a non stick, non fluffy dressing lightly over the burn	→	This helps protect from infection.
Elevate the burn	→	This reduces swelling.
Monitor the casualty	→	Check for shock and manage immediately. Check pulse and breathing.

DISLOCATION

DEFINITION

This is a joint injury in which the bones are partially or completely pulled out of position.

CAUSES

Dislocation occurs as a result of direct violence or muscle contraction.

RECOGNITION

There may be a history of injury having taken place and swelling or bruising at the joint, as well as pain. There may also be deformity or shortening of a limb and loss of movement or power.

RESPONSE

➕ A dislocation is managed in the same way as a fracture, by immobilising the joint.

➕ Dislocation may be associated with torn ligaments. Consequences may be severe, resulting in paralysis if major nerves are damaged. *No attempt should ever be made to replace the dislocation.*

SPRAINS AND STRAINS

DEFINITION

Sprains and strains are injuries to the soft tissues surrounding bones and joints.

A strain involves muscles and tendons. Tendons are fibrous cords joining muscle to bone or muscle to muscle. They are strong but inelastic.

A sprain involves ligaments. Ligaments are tough, fibrous and partially elastic tissue. They bind bone ends together in joints. They also support internal organs.

SPRAINS AND STRAINS *(continued)*

CAUSES

Injury happens when overstretching or violent and sudden movement takes place. Ankle injury often occurs when the ankle is turned outwards during slipping and tripping.

RECOGNITION

There is pain, swelling, bruising and restriction of movement.

RESPONSE

The first aid for both sprains and strains can be remembered by using the word RICE.

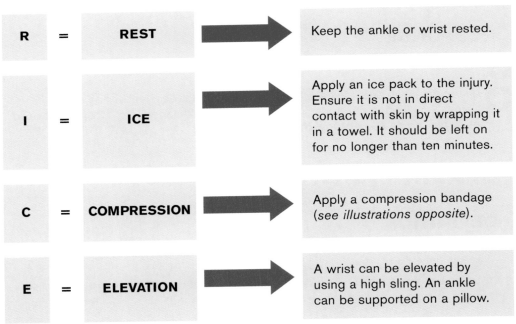

R	=	**REST**	→	Keep the ankle or wrist rested.
I	=	**ICE**	→	Apply an ice pack to the injury. Ensure it is not in direct contact with skin by wrapping it in a towel. It should be left on for no longer than ten minutes.
C	=	**COMPRESSION**	→	Apply a compression bandage (*see illustrations opposite*).
E	=	**ELEVATION**	→	A wrist can be elevated by using a high sling. An ankle can be supported on a pillow.

➕ A sprained wrist should be supported with a compression bandage. This also helps to reduce swelling. The bandage should be placed from the base of the fingers to the elbow, i.e. the joints below and above the injury. The circulation to the fingers should be monitored.

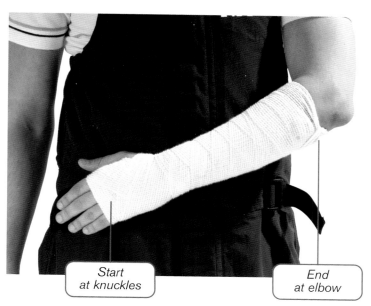

Start at knuckles

End at elbow

➕ A compression bandage on an ankle should be placed from the base of the toes to the knee, i.e. from the joint below to the joint above the injury. The foot should always be held at a 90° angle. If swelling of the ankle does not allow this, a bandage should not be applied. The circulation to the toes should be monitored.

End bandage at knee

Foot at 90° angle to leg

Start bandage at base of foot

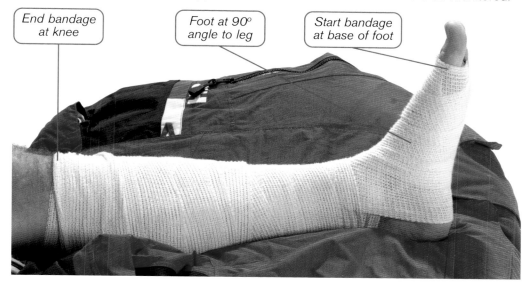

IMMOBILISATION

LOWER LIMBS AND PELVIS

A leg injury can be immobilised by using the good leg as a splint. This can be done simply using triangular bandages from the first aid kit. Any rope will also do the job just as well. The method shown (see illustration) may be used to immobilise injuries of the lower or upper leg and also to restrict movement where a fracture of the pelvis is suspected.

Commercially available splints for the leg are available, but tend to be bulky, and would take up too much space on board a small yacht to be carried as part of the emergency kit.

➕ Place padding between the ankles at the inner bony part, to prevent them rubbing together. Slide the bandage under the hollow that can be found beneath the ankle. Wrap it around the feet in a figure of eight, as shown, and tie the knot on the side of the foot opposite the injury.

➕ This tie alone will prevent a lot of leg movement and should always be the first tie placed. Shoes can be left on if the foot is not injured but laces should be loosened.

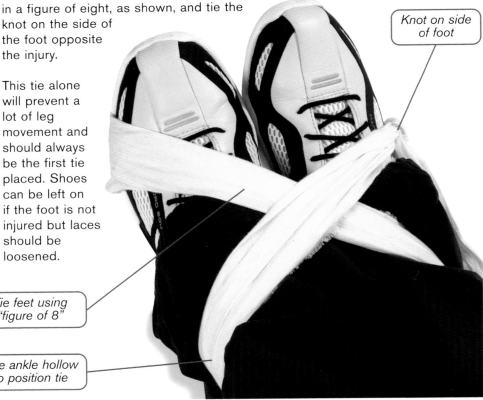

Knot on side of foot

Tie feet using "figure of 8"

Use ankle hollow to position tie

➕ Place padding between the knees and in the gaps between the legs. Rather than using bandages for this, padding can be provided by folding a towel and placing it ankle to groin.

➕ Triangular bandages should be placed as shown in the illustration. The hollows under knees and ankles should be used, and the ties then slid up or down into position.

Position ties in place

Tie feet first

Padding between legs

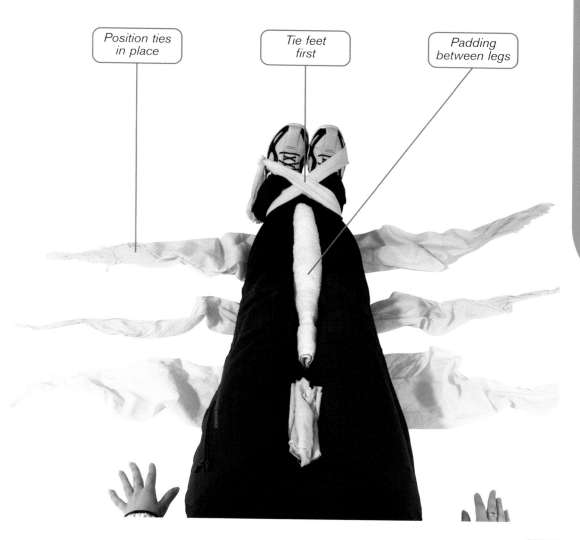

IMMOBILISATION *(continued)*

✚ All knots should be placed on the side opposite the injury. Padding may be used under the knot to make it more comfortable for the casualty. Ties should be placed at the level of the joints immediately above and below the injury (e.g. knee and ankle for a lower leg injury). Additional ties should then be placed immediately above and below the actual injury. You may use as many ties as required to secure the injury, as long as they are never placed directly over any injury.

✚ If there is bleeding at the fracture site, any dressing should be secured using a similar method of placing the triangular bandages. The legs should never be raised to place encircling bandages.

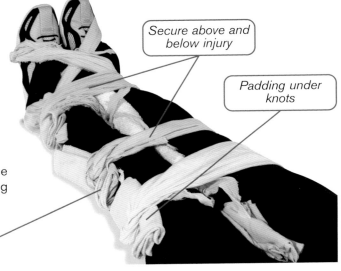

Secure above and below injury

Padding under knots

Knots on opposite side to injury

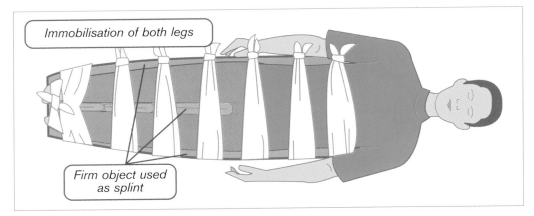

Immobilisation of both legs

Firm object used as splint

✚ If both legs are injured, a support may be placed between the legs or at the outer edge of the legs before the ties are done. Any long, firm item found on board will do (e.g. the handle of a deck brush).

SLINGS

Slings are used to support, immobilise or elevate injuries. They are used on upper and lower arm injuries, but may also be used to manage injuries affecting the collarbone, chest and shoulder.

Slings can be used in a number of different ways. They can be made using the simple triangular bandage found in the first aid box, a commercially available product, the casualty's clothing or other equipment.

The two main types of sling are the high (or elevation) sling and the low (or broad) sling.

THE LOW SLING

The low sling is used to support and immobilise shoulder, elbow, upper arm and lower arm injuries. It may also be useful where ribs are broken, to remove the weight and movement of the arm.

➕ Start by placing the fabric of the triangular bandage underneath the arm, with the long edge of the triangle placed down the body and the point towards the elbow. Lift the lower edge of the fabric up over the arm and tie in a knot at the back of the neck.

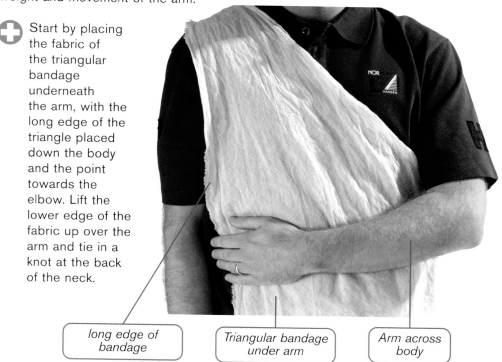

long edge of bandage

Triangular bandage under arm

Arm across body

➕ On completion, the lower arm and hand should be well supported within the sling, with the elbow held at 90°. The fingers should be accessible so that circulation can be checked. Padding may be required under the knot at the neck to make it more comfortable.

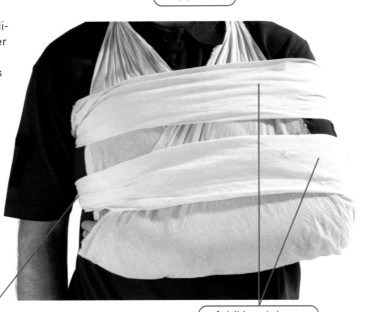

Lower arm horizontal

Fingers free to check circulation

Hand fully supported

➕ To achieve immobilisation of a shoulder joint, once the basic low sling has been applied, triangular bandages can be used to secure the arm to the body. Padding should be placed between the arm and the body for comfort.

Secure with knot opposite injury

Additional ties to stop movement

THE HIGH SLING

The high sling is used to elevate the hand and lower arm to control swelling or bleeding. It may also be used when the collar-bone is fractured.

✚ Before placing the sling, tie a knot at the point of the triangular bandage. This will allow the elbow and arm to be well supported without the need for a safety pin.

✚ Place the hand up at shoulder height and put the fabric of the triangular bandage over the arm with the long edge of the triangle placed down the body and the knotted point tucked under the elbow.

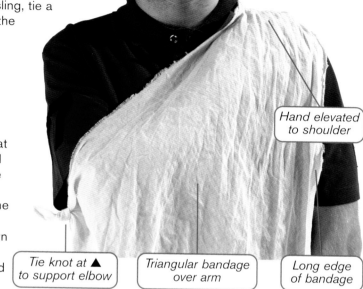

Hand elevated to shoulder

Tie knot at ▲ to support elbow

Triangular bandage over arm

Long edge of bandage

✚ Hold the elbow knot in place and support the arm. Tuck the bandage under the raised arm, making sure the hand and fingers are well enclosed.

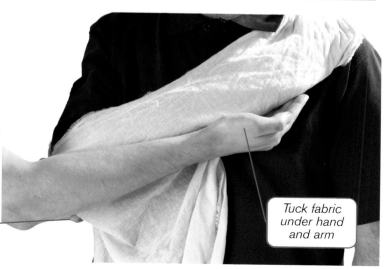

Support elbow

Tuck fabric under hand and arm

IMMOBILISATION *(continued)*

✚ Continue by taking the lower end of the triangular bandage under the elbow and around the back of the casualty, keeping the fabric as low as possible under the shoulder blade. Secure the two ends with a knot.

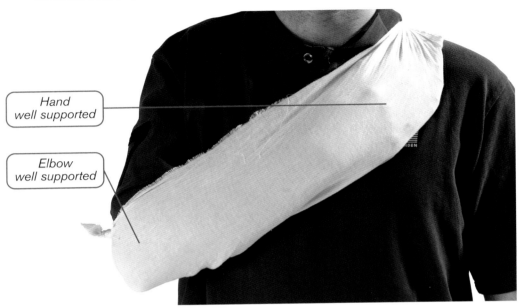

Hand
well supported

Elbow
well supported

✚ On completion, the elbow and arm should be well supported and the hand enclosed. Access to the fingers is still possible, to check the circulation.

THE IMPROVISED SLING

➕ A sling may be improvised by using the casualty's clothing to support the arm.

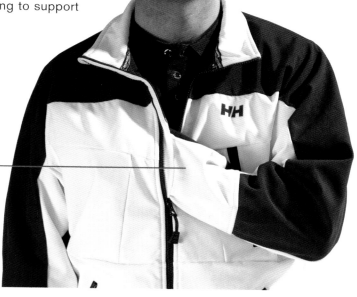

Secure arm inside clothing

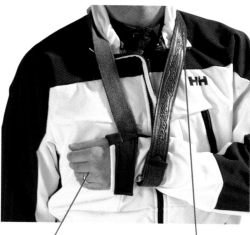

Belt used to support arm

Pad around neck for comfort

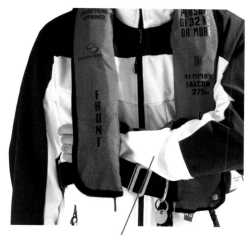

Arm supported in life jacket

IMMOBILISATION *(continued)*

➕ When immobilisation of an injured arm or shoulder cannot be achieved using a sling, it should be splinted to the body.

➕ Padding should be placed between the arm and the body. The arm is then secured to the body using triangular bandages, making sure they are never placed directly over any injury.

➕ This type of immobilisation can be improvised by using any rope or belt etc to secure the arm to the body.

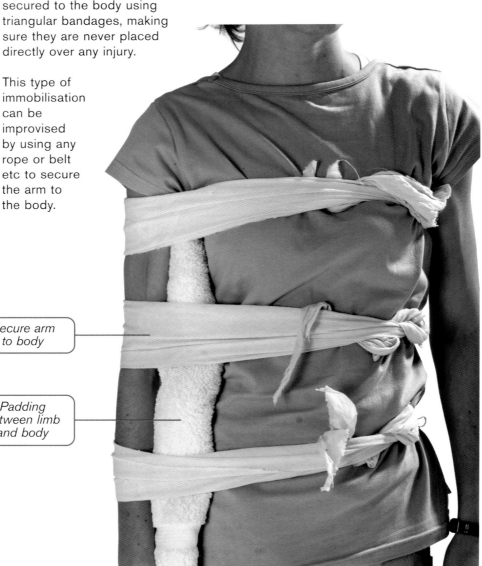

Secure arm to body

Padding between limb and body

EYE INJURY

CAUSE

Eye injuries may occur as a result of a foreign body, a chemical splash, direct trauma or a burn.

RECOGNITION

There will be a history of injury as well as evidence that can include pain, disturbance of vision, redness and swelling around the eye, inability to open the eye, copious watering of the eye, light sensitivity, visible wounds and a gritty sensation.

RESPONSE

Casualties with eye injuries are always frightened of blindness as a result of the injury, so reassuring them is a vital part of their care.

✚ The eye should be washed for a minimum of ten minutes. If a chemical splash has caused the injury, the eye needs to be washed for a minimum of 20 minutes. The washing should be done from the centre of the face outwards, to prevent contamination of the good eye and, in the case of a chemical, to prevent further contact with the skin as well as the eye.

✚ The eye should then be covered with a pad. The casualty may be shocked and should be laid down with their head and shoulders slightly raised.

✚ First aid kits contain pads shaped for use on the eye but any pad and bandage may be used to cover the affected eye once it has been washed out. Radio help should always be sought once first aid has been carried out.

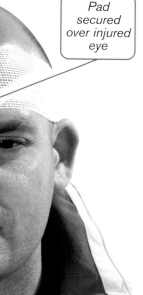

Pad secured over injured eye

HEAD INJURY

RECOGNITION

When a head injury happens, the brain is shaken up inside the skull and swelling of the brain or bleeding may occur. Any head injury is potentially serious and may result in impaired consciousness. The bony skull may be fractured and facial injuries may be present. A blow to the head may also result in neck injury.

Mild swelling of the brain results in **concussion**. The casualty may have dizziness, nausea, loss of memory, headache and brief or partial loss of consciousness. This is a temporary condition and will only last a short time.

Compression is a serious condition requiring urgent medical help. It may appear soon after injury, or it may be delayed. The most noticeable sign will be a deterioration in the level of consciousness. There will be a history of injury, intense headache, slow noisy breathing, a slow strong pulse and unequal pupils.

RESPONSE

The first aider will assess any casualty who has had a head injury for possible signs of compression. The casualty must be monitored closely over a period of time. *(See General Casualty Assessment from page 13.)* The position of the casualty will be determined by their level of consciousness. If they are unconscious, they will need to be placed in the recovery position. If they are shocked, they should be placed in the shock position but with the head and shoulders slightly raised and, if conscious, sitting propped up. If a neck injury is suspected, the spinal position should be used. *(See Spinal Injury on page 69.)*

When the base of the skull is fractured, bloodstained sticky fluid may be leaking from the ears or nose. A dressing should be placed over the ear and if the casualty becomes unconsciousness they should be placed with that ear facing down towards the deck.

A QUICK GUIDE TO HEAD INJURY MANAGEMENT

Position the casualty 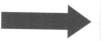 Conscious? Unconscious? Possible neck injury?

Check level of consciousness *See "AVPU" in General Casualty Assessment on page 14.*

Check pupils Are they equal in size? Do they both react to light?

Check breathing and pulse Is the pulse strong and bounding? Is the breathing slow and noisy?

Dress any wound 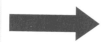 Don't apply pressure if a skull fracture is suspected.

Check for leakage from nose or ears 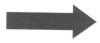 Apply dressing pad if leakage is visible.

Get help If the casualty shows signs of compression it is vital that help is sought without delay, as urgent evacuation will be required.

CHEST INJURY

RECOGNITION

An injury to the chest may be **closed** or **open**.

There will be a history of a blow to the chest. Bruising may be present. Breathing may be difficult and this will affect the casualty's skin colour, which may be pale or even blue tinged. This is due to a lack of oxygen. If the casualty coughs, you should note whether they cough up blood.

In an **open** chest injury there will be a wound to the chest. If this is deep enough to penetrate into the chest cavity, air will be going in and out of it. This will be heard as a sucking noise. There will also be frothing up of any bleeding at the wound.

RESPONSE

✚ The only difference between the care of a casualty with an open chest injury and one with a closed chest injury is the management of the sucking chest wound. The wound should initially be covered by a hand. The casualty may be able to do this while you get the first aid kit. A very specific type of dressing needs to be used. It must not stick to the wound and should be sealed down on three sides only, leaving the lower edge open. This creates a one way valve and allows air in the chest cavity to escape while preventing more air from getting into the hole.

✚ A conscious casualty should be sat upright, leaning against something for support. A shocked casualty should be placed in the shock position but with head and shoulders raised. An unconscious casualty should be placed in the recovery position, injured side down.

✚ Whichever position is required, the casualty should always be tilted over towards the side of the injury. This leaves the undamaged lung uppermost and able to expand, so aiding breathing. It also helps to keep any blood in the injured side rather than moving it to the other side and compromising the good lung.

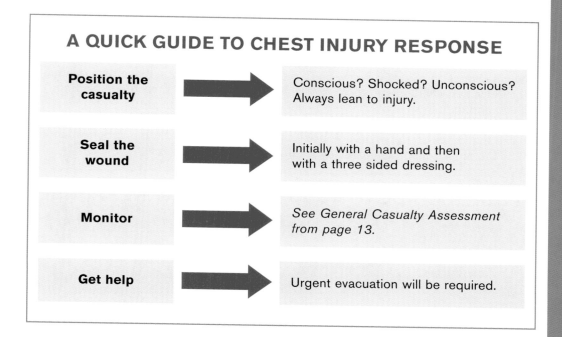

A QUICK GUIDE TO CHEST INJURY RESPONSE

Position the casualty	Conscious? Shocked? Unconscious? Always lean to injury.
Seal the wound	Initially with a hand and then with a three sided dressing.
Monitor	*See General Casualty Assessment from page 13.*
Get help	Urgent evacuation will be required.

ABDOMINAL INJURY

RECOGNITION

An injury to the abdomen may be **closed** or **open**. On examination of the abdomen, bruising and redness may be seen, or there may be no marks on the skin at all. Although the injury may appear not to be serious, it is possible there may be damage to internal organs and internal bleeding. The only sign of this will be that the casualty becomes shocked. In an **open** injury, there is a visible wound. This may be deep enough to penetrate into the abdominal cavity and its contents may be seen. In severe open injury, bowel may even be visible externally.

ABDOMINAL INJURY *(continued)*

RESPONSE

A non fluffy sterile dressing dampened by clean warm water or sterile eye wash solution should be placed over exposed bowel and held lightly in place by a bandage or cling film wrapped around the casualty. No firm dressing or pressure should be applied and the bowel should never be handled.

Raising the knees up to create a **W position** relieves pressure on the abdomen and will be the most comfortable position for the casualty.

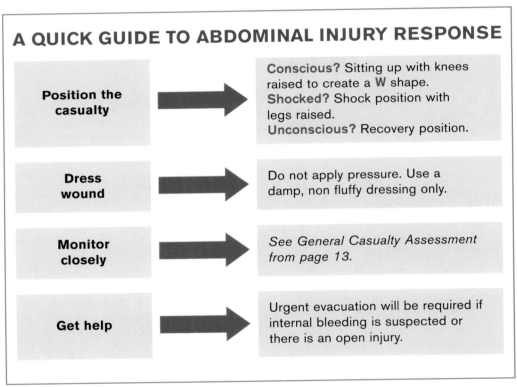

A QUICK GUIDE TO ABDOMINAL INJURY RESPONSE

Position the casualty	**Conscious?** Sitting up with knees raised to create a **W** shape. **Shocked?** Shock position with legs raised. **Unconscious?** Recovery position.
Dress wound	Do not apply pressure. Use a damp, non fluffy dressing only.
Monitor closely	*See General Casualty Assessment from page 13.*
Get help	Urgent evacuation will be required if internal bleeding is suspected or there is an open injury.

SPINAL INJURY

The spine is a series of linked small bones called vertebrae, which have flexible joints and form a long hollow tube from the base of the skull to the lower back. Enclosed in this tube is the spinal cord, which transmits messages to and from the brain. Damage to the spinal cord may result in paralysis or even death.

CAUSE

Spinal injury is caused by an abnormal force or violent twisting or bending. The most vulnerable areas are the neck and lower back. Injury may involve bones, discs, muscles, ligaments, the spinal cord and nerves (the most serious).

RECOGNITION

The most important indicator of spinal injury is the mechanism of the injury, i.e. how it occurred. Where there has been a blow to the head or a fall from a height, neck (cervical spine) injury should always be suspected. A fall from a height, jumping from a height and landing on the feet, or a blow to the back, may result in injury lower down the spine. Diving or jumping into water may also result in spine injury.

There may be pain at the spine or elsewhere, tenderness over the spine and an irregular position. Movement may be affected, with weakness or loss of control. Sensations such as burning, tingling and heaviness may be felt. There may be difficulty in breathing. Loss of bladder and bowel control may also be present.

RESPONSE

Immobilisation of the spine and maintenance of the neck in neutral alignment are the objectives for the first aider. How this is achieved will depend on the resources, equipment and manpower that are available on board. On a small yacht, it is unlikely there will be sufficient manpower or equipment to do anything other than maintain the immobilisation of the casualty by holding their head still.

It is vital that medical advice is sought, as urgent evacuation will be required. On rescue, the emergency services will provide a neck collar and special immobilising stretchers in order to be able to move the casualty safely. A neck collar alone does not prevent head movement. You should not attempt to make a collar from rolled up materials. This will not immobilise the neck and you may cause harm in the attempt. Always wait for instructions from medical help.

SPINAL INJURY *(continued)*

➕ Ensure it is safe to approach the casualty. Assess if the casualty has a clear airway and is breathing. It is vital to tell the casualty not to move.

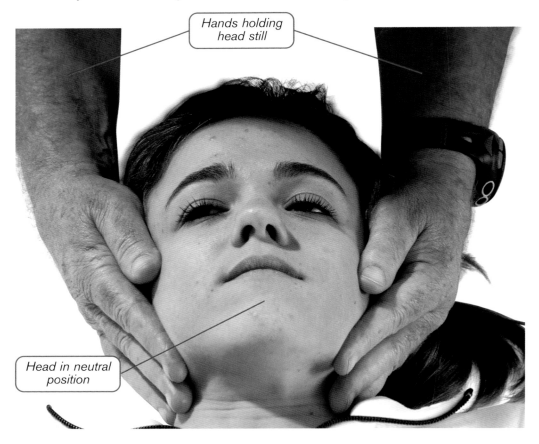

Hands holding head still

Head in neutral position

➕ The rescuer should support the casualty's head in a neutral position and keep the casualty from making any movement. This may be done by placing the hands on either side of their head as shown in the illustration above.

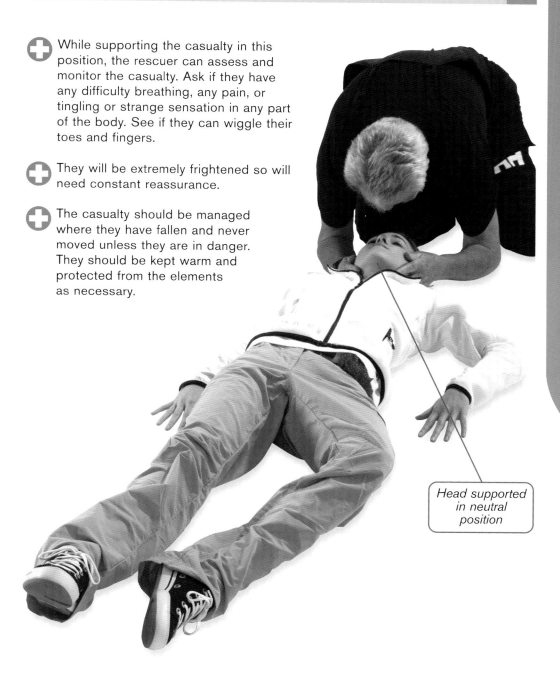

➕ While supporting the casualty in this position, the rescuer can assess and monitor the casualty. Ask if they have any difficulty breathing, any pain, or tingling or strange sensation in any part of the body. See if they can wiggle their toes and fingers.

➕ They will be extremely frightened so will need constant reassurance.

➕ The casualty should be managed where they have fallen and never moved unless they are in danger. They should be kept warm and protected from the elements as necessary.

Head supported in neutral position

SPINAL INJURY *(continued)*

✚ If the casualty becomes unconscious, the priority changes to protecting their airway. This means the casualty must be placed in the recovery position. If there are other people on board, they can assist with the positioning of the casualty but the casualty's head should always be held and their neck supported. The person doing this will be the one in charge and giving instructions. No one should do anything to the casualty until they are given the go ahead by the rescuer supporting the head.

✚ If you are alone with the casualty, carry out the recovery position in the usual way but make sure the head is well supported when you turn the casualty and do not let the head drop to the deck but keep the spine from the neck down as straight as possible.

This chapter details
conditions related to
the environment at sea
and the weather conditions
to which a yachtsman may
be exposed.

- Seasickness

- Heat Exhaustion

- Heatstroke

- Sunburn

- Hypothermia

- Frostbite

- Immersion Foot

ENVIRONMENTAL
INJURY

SEASICKNESS

Seasickness can affect the most experienced yachtsman and it may happen even in relatively calm waters. As well as the obvious physical symptoms, anxiety is also a feature of seasickness.

Seasickness will prevent crew from carrying out tasks on board and can affect safety. It is important to treat it as a serious issue.

Seeing and hearing another person vomiting can cause others on board to become ill.

RECOGNITION

The casualty starts to feel sluggish and unwell, and begins to feel nauseous. This leads on to vomiting. Vomiting does not relieve the symptoms and the casualty will want to lie down. Women are more likely to suffer seasickness at the time of their monthly period.

PREVENTION

It helps to be prepared for the journey. There are medicines for seasickness, in the form of tablets or skin patches, and these need to be taken before departure. Some are available as over the counter remedies, while others may need to be obtained from a doctor on prescription. It is always important to follow the instructions for their use. Medicines work on the body in different ways and if one medicine appears not to help it is always worth changing to another. As well as medicines, there are methods based on acupressure, and even hypnosis has been tried to cure seasickness. One old fashioned tried and tested remedy is to eat ginger.

Avoiding a hangover from the farewell party before a trip will also help!

RESPONSE

If someone is feeling nauseated and wobbly, they may still be able to carry out tasks on board. As the seasickness progresses to vomiting, however, they will probably want to lie down. Let them rest down below, making sure they keep that bucket close by. They may very well sleep.

It is not a good idea for an unsteady person to vomit over the side of the yacht, as they could overbalance and fall in to the sea. A bucket should always be used.

HEAT EXHAUSTION

DEFINITION

Heat exhaustion occurs when there is loss of salt and water from the body, resulting in circulatory collapse.

CAUSE

Fluid loss may come from excessive diarrhoea and vomiting, or from sweating, which is the primary cause. This is seen in hot, humid climates, especially when the casualty is not acclimatised

RECOGNITION

Despite its name, in heat exhaustion the casualty is not hot. Their body temperature is normal. They have pale, cold, clammy skin, as in shock, and also have fast, shallow breathing and a rapid, weak pulse.

Fatigue, weakness and muscle cramps are present. There is headache, giddiness and possibly fainting, with mood changes and mental deterioration. The casualty is dehydrated, but it should be noted that thirst is a late sign of dehydration.

RESPONSE

The casualty should be kept in a cool environment and laid down with their legs elevated, as in shock. They should be given fluids to replace the fluids that have been lost but should avoid gulping as this may lead to vomiting. Do not give the casualty salt to replace the salt that has been lost, as this may cause vomiting.

Medical advice should be sought, as heat exhaustion may lead to the more serious condition of heatstroke.

HEATSTROKE

DEFINITION

There is a failure of the body's "thermostat" to control body temperature by sweating, allowing the body to overheat, with the body temperature rising to over 40°C.

CAUSE

Heatstroke can follow on from heat exhaustion that has not been recognised or managed well. A feverish illness can also lead to heatstroke. Working in an environment that is hot and humid, and that does not allow natural body cooling by sweating to take place, may also result in heatstroke.

RECOGNITION

The casualty feels hot to the touch and is flushed red, and their skin is dry because they are not sweating. They will initially be restless and complaining of dizziness and headache. This will progress to delirium, coma and death. The pulse is strong and bounding, while breathing is noisy.

RESPONSE

✚ The response needs to be rapid and must commence before medical help arrives.

✚ Keep the casualty in the cool and out of the sun. Take off all their clothes and cover them with a wet sheet. Soaking a sheet in sea water is the easiest way to do this. If the casualty is unconscious or very drowsy, they should be placed in the recovery position.

✚ The body heat from the casualty causes the moisture to evaporate from the sheet and leads to cooling. This mimics the effect of sweating.

✚ It is imperative that you seek emergency medical help as soon as possible, as the casualty will need urgent evacuation. Until the casualty is conscious again and able to drink, there will be no way to replace lost fluid as the necessary equipment is unlikely to be available on a small yacht.

✚ Monitor the casualty's pulse, breathing and consciousness at ten minute intervals.

SUNBURN

CAUSE

A breeze at sea may keep you cool, but there is more likelihood of you being exposed to sunlight and burning at sea than ashore. This can happen without you noticing.

PREVENTION

A strong sun block should always be used on exposed skin, and protective clothing worn. Children should always be protected by total block.

RECOGNITION

Sunburn is actually a heat burn *(see pages 43-45)* caused by radiation. It may cause redness and tenderness only (superficial burn) or blister (partial thickness burn).

RESPONSE

✚ Treat sunburn as you would treat any burn, by cooling it. Blisters should never be burst. Proprietary brands of after sun cooling lotion are available. These contain a cooling agent and are suitable for use on superficial burns. Simple pain relief, such as paracetamol or ibuprofen, will also help with comfort.

✚ The casualty may also be suffering from heat exhaustion and this should be treated. They should drink plenty of fluids.

HYPOTHERMIA

DEFINITION

Hypothermia is when the core body temperature drops below 35°C.

CAUSES

Hypothermia may happen after immersion in cold water or exposure in a cold environment. Certain medical conditions and poor diet may also be contributing factors, as can be the effects of alcohol or drugs.

HYPOTHERMIA *(continued)*

RECOGNITION

Initially, the casualty feels cold and miserable. Their skin feels cold and may look pale. Shivering is the body's attempt to keep warm, but this sign disappears as the casualty's body temperature drops. Muscles are affected, with poor coordination and slurred speech. The casualty's behaviour becomes confused and irrational. Their level of consciousness deteriorates rapidly, leading to unconsciousness. Their pulse and breathing gradually slow down until they cannot be detected. Without intervention, hypothermia will eventually lead to death.

RESPONSE

➕ The casualty should be removed from the cold environment. The main treatment is to slowly rewarm the casualty. This may be done in a number of ways, depending on their condition.

➕ If a casualty is rescued from the water, they should preferably be kept horizontal. Once on board, they should be manhandled as little as possible.

➕ Remove the casualty's wet clothing. On a small yacht where warm baths are not available, you can rewarm the person by putting them to bed and warming them with blankets. Rewarming should be slow and passive. Do not rub the casualty's skin or use hot water bottles. If they are conscious and able to drink safely, the casualty should be given warm drinks.

➕ One way to rewarm someone is known as the buddy system. The rescuer, wearing only light clothes, climbs into the bed or sleeping bag with the casualty and warms them with their own body heat.

FROSTBITE

DEFINITION

Frostbite is a cold injury in a localised area on the extremities, usually the hands, feet, nose and ears.

RECOGNITION

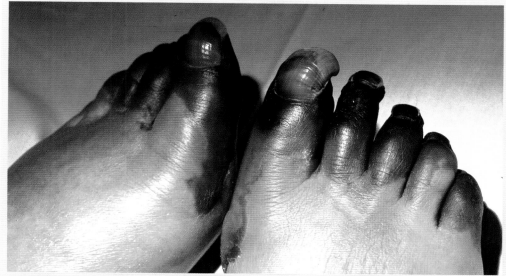

The skin may be white and waxy or blistered black and blue where all the tissue is frozen and dead.

RESPONSE

The treatment for frostbite is the same as for a cold burn *(see pages 45-46)*. Warm the damaged tissue slowly and gently. Hands or feet may be immersed in warm water kept at about 40°C. The affected part should then be dressed with a non stick, non fluffy dressing and be well padded. Hands should be kept elevated in a sling. If a foot is affected, the casualty should be resting in a bunk with the foot elevated. Pain relief will be needed. Medical advice should be sought.

IMMERSION FOOT

This condition develops when the feet are cold and wet for long periods. It is also known as trench foot. The feet become white as circulation reduces, and the tissues become numb and swollen.

 Dry the feet gently and warm them but do not rub the skin. Attention should be paid to keeping feet and footwear as dry as possible and socks should be changed daily.

This chapter deals with illness that may need to be dealt with as an emergency and involve the evacuation of a casualty, as well as illness that can be managed on board.

- Chest Pain

- Seizures

- Diabetes

- Asthma

- Poisoning

- Bites and Stings

ILLNESS AND MEDICAL EMERGENCIES

CHEST PAIN

CAUSE

Disease of the cardiovascular system may be slow and progressive, often with no external signs or symptoms until illness suddenly presents. It is a major cause of death in the Western world.

When the blood vessels supplying blood to the heart become narrowed or blocked, the supply of oxygen to the heart muscle is affected. This results in pain.

If oxygen supplies are restricted because of a partial blockage, the resulting pain is known as **angina** (*angina pectoris*). The pain is triggered by anything that requires the heart to beat faster, such as physical activity or emotion.

When the oxygen supply to the heart is completely cut off, heart muscle dies, resulting in pain. This is known as a **heart attack** (*myocardial infarction*).

RECOGNITION

Pain may be felt in the centre of the chest or radiate out to the left arm, jaw, back and upper abdomen.

In angina, the pain generally goes when the casualty is at rest, but it does recur. The casualty may be breathless, pale and sweaty, and feels weak.

Heart attack pain is sudden and is not triggered by anything. It persists, and does not go when the casualty is at rest. The casualty may have difficulty breathing and be pale in colour or blue tinged (*cyanosis*). They may have nausea and vomiting, they may be sweating and their pulse may be irregular, weak, and fast. Heart attack casualties sometimes describe experiencing a sense of doom.

RESPONSE

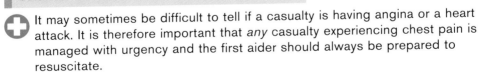
It may sometimes be difficult to tell if a casualty is having angina or a heart attack. It is therefore important that *any* casualty experiencing chest pain is managed with urgency and the first aider should always be prepared to resuscitate.

QUICK GUIDE TO MANAGING CHEST PAIN

Position the casualty Position the casualty on the deck, sitting up well supported, and loosen their clothing. This will aid breathing.

Be prepared to resuscitate The casualty may have a cardiac arrest at any time. From the sitting position on the deck, it is easier to lay them flat to commence resuscitation.

Get help It is vital that radio emergency help is sought immediately.

Assist the casualty to take their own angina medication if they have it 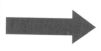 This medication dilates blood vessels, improving the flow of oxygen to the heart. It is absorbed from the mouth straight into the bloodstream, so works quickly.

If pain persists, give the casualty one aspirin tablet to chew and keep in the mouth 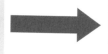 The aspirin tablet must be broken up and kept in the mouth, under the tongue. It is quickly absorbed and reduces blood clotting. Do not give aspirin to an asthmatic or someone who has a known aspirin allergy.

Monitor the casualty Closely monitor the casualty. Count their pulse rate and note if it is irregular. Note the casualty's breathing rate and skin colour.

SEIZURES

DEFINITION

Seizures are sometimes called fits or convulsions. They involve the involuntary contraction of the muscles due to a disturbance of electrical activity in the brain.

CAUSE

There are a number of causes of seizures, including epilepsy, head injury, poisoning, alcohol, lack of oxygen (hypoxia), low blood sugar (hypoglycaemia), infection and high temperature.

RECOGNITION

If someone on board is known to have seizures, they should ensure they have sufficient medication with them. They should also tell other crew so that everyone is aware of their medical condition and knows what to do to help, should they have a seizure.

Seizures can vary from involving the whole body to only parts of it. Some casualties just lose awareness of their surroundings. Some epileptics are aware of when they are about to have a seizure, experiencing a warning known as an aura, and can prepare for it.

RESPONSE

The rescuer cannot stop the seizure from happening. Their role is to make sure the casualty is not in danger while the seizure is happening and to look after them during the recovery phase.

No attempt should ever be made to restrain the casualty while they are fitting, or to put anything into their mouth.

QUICK GUIDE TO MANAGING SEIZURES

Protect the casualty from dangers 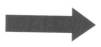 No attempt should be made to restrain a casualty or put anything in their mouth during the seizure. Remove items around the casualty to make the area safer.

Note the extent and duration of seizure 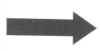 Seizures can vary from involving the whole body to only parts of it. Some casualties just lose awareness of their surroundings.

Get help If the fitting does not stop, it is vital to get help immediately from radio medical advice. Advice should also be sought if this is the first time a casualty has experienced a seizure.

When the seizure stops The casualty may be unconscious and should be placed in the recovery position until they are awake. They should be monitored like any unconscious casualty.

After the seizure The casualty will be very tired and may want to sleep. Having a seizure can be exhausting.

Monitor the casualty 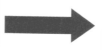 Closely monitor the casualty. Count their pulse rate and breathing rate. If still unconscious, their breathing should be checked every one to two minutes and their level of consciousness should also be assessed.

DIABETES

In diabetes (the full name is diabetes mellitus), the body is unable to regulate sugar levels in the body. This condition may be controlled by diet, oral medication or insulin injection, depending on its type and severity.

When blood sugar levels fall too low, the diabetic is said to be hypoglycaemic or "hypo". This may happen very quickly and will lead rapidly to unconsciousness. It may also occur in the non diabetic casualty, for example after a fit or an alcohol binge.

When blood sugar is raised, the diabetic is said to be hyperglycaemic. This may also lead to the casualty becoming unconscious but in this case it does not happen suddenly, but the casualty's condition gradually worsens until they become unconscious. This may be accompanied by a distinctive smell on the breath (*ketones*) similar to nail varnish remover or pear drops.

RECOGNITION OF HYPOGLYCAEMIA

The casualty's behaviour changes and they may become aggressive and uncooperative. Their level of consciousness will fall and their skin will be sweaty.

RESPONSE

✚ If the casualty is hypoglycaemic, this needs to be managed before they become unconscious. The treatment is to get sugar into them. Give them a milky drink with lots of sugar added, or get them to eat a chocolate bar or even sugar lumps until they start to feel normal again.

✚ If the casualty is too drowsy to eat or drink, or has actually become unconscious, smear jam or honey around the inside of their mouth and gums. The sugar will be absorbed through the mouth tissue straight into the bloodstream.

✚ When a hypoglycaemic casualty is unconscious, they will need sugar to be given in an injectable format straight into a vein. This is a medical emergency and medical help will be needed. The casualty should be placed in the recovery position while awaiting help.

✚ A diabetic person may bring high sugar sweets on board with them and always keep them at hand so they are ready to use.

ASTHMA

CAUSE

In asthma, there is constriction and inflammation of the airway passages, making it difficult for air to pass through them. This results in the casualty making a wheezing sound as they breathe.

There is no common cause of asthma. Contributing factors to an asthma attack (known as triggers) may include allergies, pollution, exercise, drugs, temperature changes, respiratory infection, stress and emotion. Those suffering from asthma may know what their triggers are and take steps to avoid them.

Asthma attacks may also be triggered by some over the counter medicines. Beware of aspirin, ibuprofen, and some seasickness remedies.

RECOGNITION

An asthma attack is very frightening for the casualty. They will be struggling to breathe, wheezing, gasping and experiencing shortness of breath. Their skin colour will reflect this and may be pale or blue around the lips. Their pulse will be fast.

RESPONSE

➕ Assist the casualty to take their medication. It is important not to crowd them as a sense of claustrophobia can cause anxiety and make their breathing worse.

➕ If a known asthmatic is to be on board, ensure they have sufficient supplies of their medication with them and that these are easily accessible on board.

QUICK GUIDE TO MANAGING AN ASTHMA ATTACK

Position the casualty in a well ventilated area 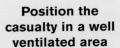	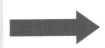	Position the casualty sitting upright. It also helps if they lean forward on a support. This expands the chest cavity and assists with breathing. Keep the casualty away from potential triggers.
Reassure the casualty		Anxiety will make the attack worse and constant reassurance is vital.
Assist the casualty to take their own medication if they have it		This medication dilates the air tubes and is known as a reliever. It is important that the casualty uses their inhaler properly and breathes the drug down into the lungs. The usual dose is one or two puffs.

"Reliever" inhaler

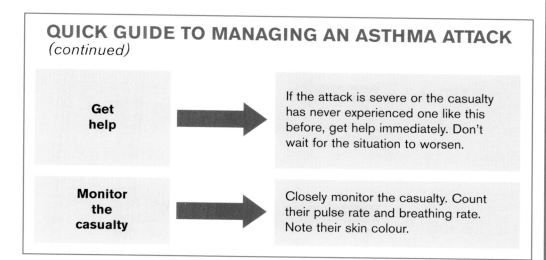

QUICK GUIDE TO MANAGING AN ASTHMA ATTACK
(continued)

Get help	If the attack is severe or the casualty has never experienced one like this before, get help immediately. Don't wait for the situation to worsen.
Monitor the casualty	Closely monitor the casualty. Count their pulse rate and breathing rate. Note their skin colour.

POISONING

DEFINITION

A poison is any substance that may cause temporary or permanent harm, and even death, when it is taken into the body in sufficient quantity. Poisons enter the body through the mouth (ingestion), by breathing them in (inhalation), through bites and stings (injection) and through the skin (absorption).

RECOGNITION

It is important to recognise the possible signs and symptoms of poisoning, so the rescuer is not put in danger as well. The casualty's level of consciousness may be altered, they may have difficulty breathing or be vomiting, and they may have burns on their skin. A clue to possible poisoning may be found in whatever the casualty was doing recently.

A QUICK GUIDE TO POISONING

ABC	Check the casualty has an airway and is breathing. If breathing is present, the casualty will have circulation.
Position the casualty	If the casualty is unconscious, put them in the recovery position. If they are shocked, lay them down with legs raised. If they are conscious but having difficulty breathing, position them sitting and propped up.
Monitor the casualty	*See casualty observation on pages 14-15.*
Find out about the poison	What has the casualty been exposed to? When? How long for?
Provide first aid	Appropriately, according to the type of poisoning.
Get help	Medical advice will need to be sought in all cases of poisoning.

A QUICK GUIDE TO TYPES OF POISONING

Swallowed poisons 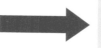 Dilute the poison by getting the casualty to sip water or milk slowly. They should stop if they feel sick. Eating ice cream will also work, and children are usually more cooperative with this method.
Vomiting may compromise the airway and if the poison was corrosive it will burn as it comes up and cause further damage.

Skin contamination Wash the poison off the skin. Remove contaminated clothing, taking care not to come into contact with it yourself.

Inhaled poison Ensure the casualty is in a well ventilated area. Monitor their breathing closely. Do not let the casualty rub their eyes.

Intentional overdose Find out what was taken, when and how much – not why. Retain any unused medicines or vomit for identification if needed.

Alcohol There is a danger of unconsciousness, vomiting and secondary injury as well as hypothermia.

Food poisoning Rest and fluids only.

BITES AND STINGS

CAUSE

Bites and stings may be from spiders, insects, snakes and marine creatures. The likelihood of these occurring depends on where the yacht is sailing and where the crew go ashore.

RECOGNITION

This will depend on the cause. There may be local reaction with pain and swelling, or an all over (systemic) reaction where there is an allergic response or severe shock.

QUICK GUIDE TO BITES AND STINGS

Insect stings

Scrape the sting off sideways, using the edge of a knife blade or even a credit card. Squeezing or using tweezers can cause any poison to get into the body.

If the sting is in a limb, elevate it to reduce swelling and apply an ice pack. If stung in the mouth, suck ice or rinse with cold water.

Snakebites

Try to identify the snake. Immobilise the limb and keep the casualty as still as possible to slow the circulation of venom around the body. Keep the bite below the level of the heart.

Sea creatures (e.g. coral, jellyfish, anemones)

Rest, ice and elevation.

Tropical jellyfish

Wash with vinegar or sea water. Immobilise the limb. Place a light compression bandage above the sting.

Marine puncture wound (e.g. weever fish, sea urchin)

Immerse in warm water. Do not bandage the wound.

Animal bite

Clean and treat like any wound. Infection is a risk and, if you are not in UK waters, consider rabies.

This chapter details how to manage life threatening situations in children.

- **Resuscitation of Children and Infants**

- **The Choking Child**

CHILDREN AND INFANTS

RESUSCITATION OF CHILDREN AND INFANTS

An infant is considered to be a child under one year old, while a child is between one year old and puberty.

Many people fear that attempting resuscitation on a child will cause harm. This fear is unfounded. A layperson who has not had special training and practice in the resuscitation of children may use the adult form (*see Chapter 2*). Minor modifications to the adult sequence make it more suitable for use in children. These are:

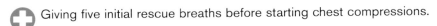 Giving five initial rescue breaths before starting chest compressions.

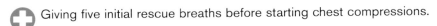 If alone, performing CPR for approximately one minute before going for help.

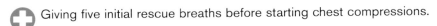 Compressing the chest by approximately one-third of its depth, using two fingers for an infant under one year and one or two hands for a child over one year as needed, to achieve an adequate depth of compression.

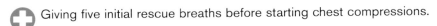 Gently stimulate the child and ask loudly, "Are you all right?"

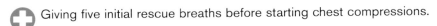 Do not shake infants or children with suspected cervical spine injury.

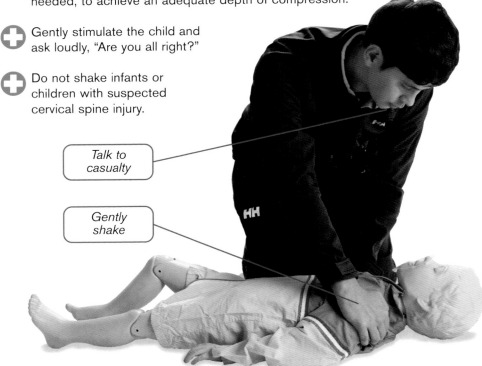

Talk to casualty

Gently shake

➕ With the child initially in the position in which they were found, place your hand on their forehead and gently tilt the head back. (*In an infant, only lift the chin.*)

➕ At the same time, with your fingertip(s) under the point of the child's chin, lift the chin. Do not push on the soft tissues under the chin as this may block the airway.

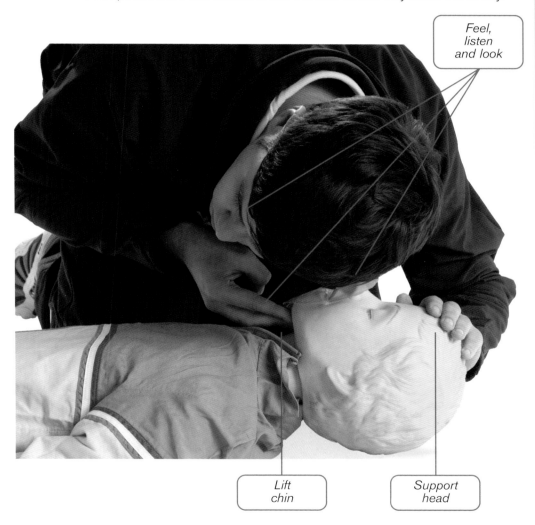

Feel, listen and look

Lift chin

Support head

RESUSCITATION OF
CHILDREN AND INFANTS *(continued)*

➕ Take a breath, and cover the mouth and nose of the child with your mouth, making sure you have a good seal. If the nose and mouth cannot both be covered in an older child, attempt a seal over either the mouth or the nose only. If using the nose, make sure the lips are closed to prevent air escaping.

➕ Blow steadily into the mouth and nose over 1–1.5 seconds, sufficient to make the chest visibly rise. Maintain head tilt and chin lift (*or chin lift only in an infant*), take your mouth away from the child, and watch for the chest to fall as air comes out.

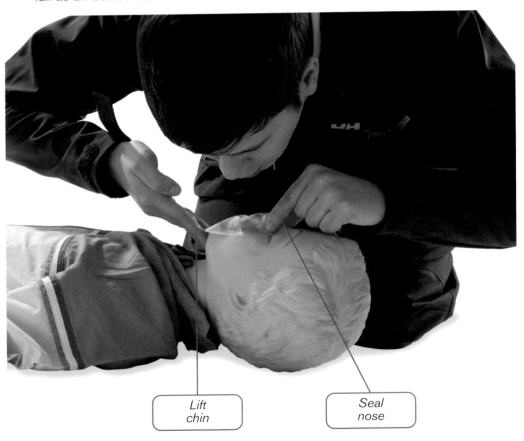

Lift chin

Seal nose

➕ Take another breath and repeat this sequence five times.

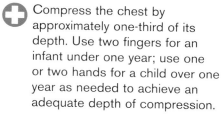 Compress the chest by approximately one-third of its depth. Use two fingers for an infant under one year; use one or two hands for a child over one year as needed to achieve an adequate depth of compression.

Do 30 compressions.

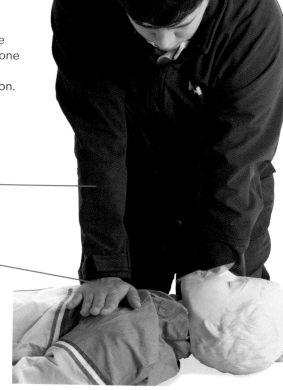

Arm straight

Heel of hand in centre of chest

Give two breaths, then continue with a sequence of 30 compressions to two breaths.

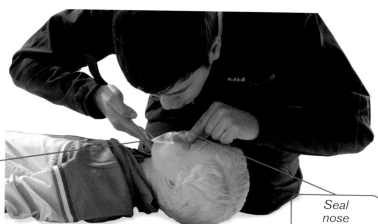

Lift chin

Seal nose

A SUMMARY OF BASIC LIFE SUPPORT FOR INFANTS AND CHILDREN

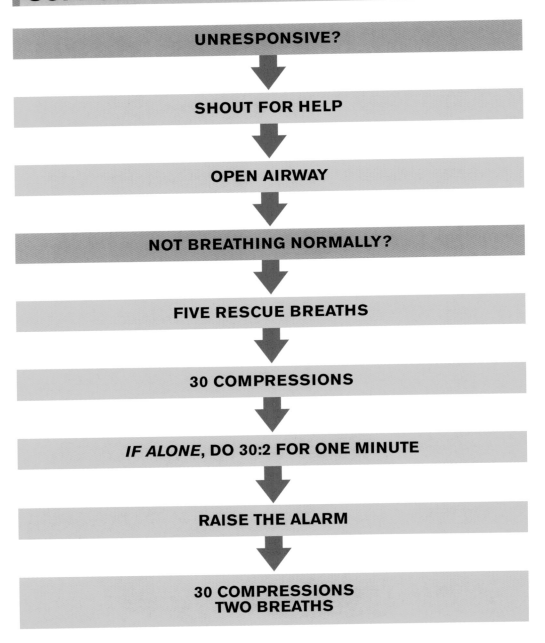

UNRESPONSIVE?

SHOUT FOR HELP

OPEN AIRWAY

NOT BREATHING NORMALLY?

FIVE RESCUE BREATHS

30 COMPRESSIONS

IF ALONE, DO 30:2 FOR ONE MINUTE

RAISE THE ALARM

30 COMPRESSIONS
TWO BREATHS

THE CHOKING CHILD

CAUSE

The majority of choking events in children occur during play or whilst eating.

THREAT

When a foreign object enters the airway, the child reacts immediately by coughing in an attempt to expel it. A spontaneous cough is likely to be more effective and safer than any manoeuvre a rescuer might perform. If coughing is absent or ineffective, and there is complete obstruction of the airway, the child will rapidly become asphyxiated.

RECOGNITION

Onset is sudden with no other signs of illness. Clues, such as symptoms appearing when the child is eating or playing with small objects, will alert the rescuer.
The incident may be witnessed.

RESPONSE

➕ If there is a sudden onset of breathing distress, perhaps with coughing or noisy breathing, and the child is able to cry or talk and take breaths, intervention is not required but the child must be monitored closely.

➕ If coughing is ineffective at clearing the airway intervention, there is no coughing or noise, the child is unable to breathe, their skin is pallid or blue and there is a decrease in consciousness, intervention is needed rapidly.

➕ Active intervention is required only when coughing becomes ineffective, but this needs to be commenced rapidly and confidently.

UNCONSCIOUS

➕ If the child is, or becomes, unconscious place them on a firm, flat surface. Do not leave the child at this stage. Commence CPR.

➕ When opening the airway, look in the mouth for any obvious object. Only if this is visible, make an attempt to remove it with a single finger sweep. Do not attempt blind or repeated finger sweeps as this may push an object further in and cause injury. Continue with CPR as previously illustrated.

THE CHOKING CHILD *(continued)*

➕ If the child regains consciousness and is breathing effectively, place them in a safe side lying (recovery) position and monitor their breathing and level of consciousness while waiting for help to arrive.

CONSCIOUS

Back slaps, and chest or abdominal thrusts, create an "artificial cough" to increase pressure in the chest and dislodge the foreign object.

CONSCIOUS INFANT (UNDER ONE YEAR OLD)

If the infant is still conscious but has absent or ineffective coughing, give back blows. If back blows do not relieve the obstruction, give chest thrusts.

Back blows	Chest thrusts
Support the infant lying on their front in a head downwards position, to enable gravity to assist removal of the foreign object.	Turn the infant onto their back into a head downwards position. This is achieved safely by placing your free arm along the infant's back and encircling the back of their head with your hand.
A seated or kneeling rescuer should be able to support the infant safely across their lap.	Support the infant down your arm, which is placed down (or across) your thigh.
Support the infant's head by placing the thumb of one hand at the angle of the lower jaw, and one or two fingers from the same hand at the same point on the other side of the jaw.	Place two fingers on the infant's lower breastbone, just above the V point where the ribs meet.
Do not compress the soft tissues under the jaw, as this will further obstruct the airway.	Deliver five chest thrusts. These are similar to chest compressions, but sharper in nature and delivered at a slower rate.
Give up to five sharp back blows with the heel of one hand in the middle of the back between the shoulder blades.	**Do not use abdominal thrusts for infants.**
The aim is to relieve the obstruction with each blow rather than to give all five blows.	

Following chest thrusts, reassess the infant. If the object has not been expelled and the child is still conscious, continue the sequence of back blows and chest thrusts.

CONSCIOUS CHILD (OVER ONE YEAR OLD)

If the child is still conscious but has absent or ineffective coughing, give back blows. If back blows do not relieve the obstruction, give abdominal thrusts.

Back blows

Back blows are more effective if the child is positioned head down.

A small child may be placed across the rescuer's lap, as with an infant.

If this is not possible, support the child in a forward leaning position and deliver the back blows from behind.

If back blows fail to dislodge the object, and the child is still conscious, use abdominal thrusts.

Abdominal thrusts

Stand or kneel behind the child. Place your arms under the child's arms and encircle their torso.

Clench your fist and place it midway between the belly button and the breastbone.

Grasp this hand with your other hand and pull sharply inwards and upwards.

Repeat up to five times.

Ensure that pressure is not applied to the lower rib cage, as this may cause abdominal trauma.

Do not use abdominal thrusts for infants.

Following abdominal thrusts, reassess the child. If the object has not been expelled and the child is still conscious, continue the sequence of back blows and abdominal thrusts.

The object may appear to be successfully expelled but part of it may remain in the airway and cause complications. Thrusts may cause internal injury. Medical assistance should always be sought.

This chapter details the movement of a casualty on board and evacuation procedures, as well as advice on first aid equipment and medicines to be carried.

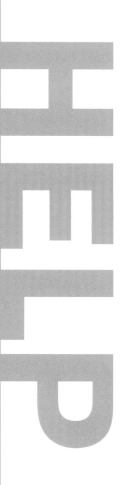

- Moving a Casualty

- Evacuation of a Casualty

- Transfer to
  Rescue Vessel

- Radio Medical Advice

- First Aid Equipment

- Medicines

- Hygiene

MOVING A CASUALTY

ON BOARD

➕ Do not move the casualty unless they are in immediate danger, as this may worsen their condition. Place them in a position appropriate to their injury and carry out assessment and treatment as needed. Once stable, they may be moved to a more suitable location on board. In a serious incident, do not move the casualty until medical advice has been sought.

➕ When moving a casualty, particularly in the small confined spaces on a yacht, you must consider personal and casualty safety, the condition of the casualty, manpower and equipment available on board, and basic principles of lifting and moving. Any move should always be planned well.

➕ Improvisation is useful. For example, a stretcher can be fashioned from jackets and dinghy oars. The oars can be placed through the jacket sleeves with jacket fronts closed around them to create the stretcher, but always test that it will take the casualty's weight before using it. Once they are on the stretcher, make sure the casualty is secured and comfortable.

➕ If the casualty is able to walk, always support them from the injured side when walking with them.

➕ If two people are attempting to carry a casualty, they should always make sure their hand grips are secure, (see illustrations).

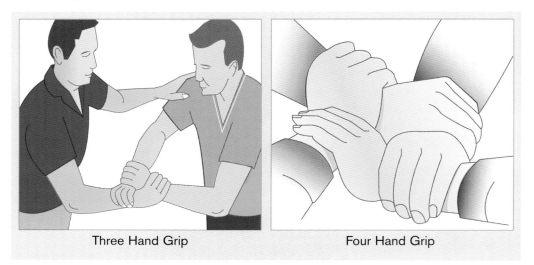

| Three Hand Grip | Four Hand Grip |

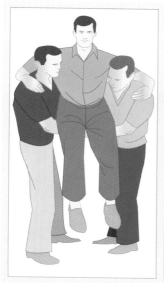 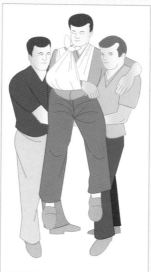 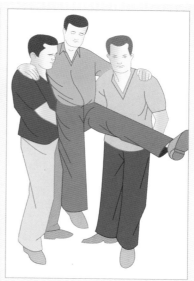

EVACUATION OF A CASUALTY

If you require medical assistance, this should be done via the coastguards (*see Radio Medical Advice on page 108*). They will liaise with rescue organisations to arrange the evacuation of the casualty as needed, and will put you in contact with radio medical advice.

HELICOPTER EVACUATION

You should closely follow the instructions given to you by the rescue helicopter. Contact with the helicopter is usually on VHF.

As well as the nature of the casualty's distress, the following information will be required by the coastguard, who will relay it to the rescue helicopter:

• Vessel identity, position, speed and course

• What radios, distress rockets or flares are on board.

EVACUATION OF A CASUALTY *(continued)*

➕ When a helicopter comes to your assistance, you should listen to the instructions given, which will include the speed and direction you should maintain. The deck should be cleared of obstacles, as far as possible, and any loose items secured. The winch wire will have a static charge and should not be touched until this has been discharged in the sea. This is achieved by the earthing wire fitted to the winch hook. The line should not be tied to the boat.

You may be asked to hang onto the line when the casualty is being winched up on a "highline" as this helps prevent them spinning in the downdraught.

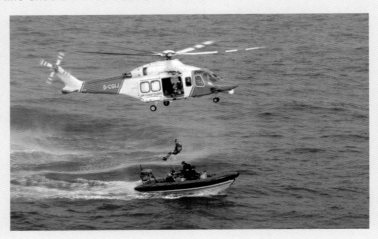

TRANSFER TO RESCUE VESSEL

➕ Keep the casualty secure on board your yacht until the rescuers come on board to assess the situation. Transferring the casualty may be a hazardous procedure and you don't want anyone ending up in the water or being injured.

RADIO MEDICAL ADVICE

Radio Medical Advice (RMA) is available free of charge to provide support in cases where an individual suffers either illness or an accident at sea. For the UK, the officially designated centres are at Queen Alexandra Hospital, Portsmouth and at Aberdeen Royal Infirmary.

To obtain radio medical advice, skippers should first contact HM Coastguard. Contact should be made on MF DSC, VHF DSC, VHF Channel 16 or INMARSAT.

Urgent calls for assistance may be broadcast using the normal Urgency pro words "PAN PAN" as follows:

"PAN PAN" (x3) "All Stations" (x3) OR individual coastguard/coast station (x3) if name is known.

"This is [yacht name]" (x3) "Call Sign ………." "In Position …….." "I require medical advice" "Over".

The coastguard or coast station will direct the caller to a working frequency, and is obliged to seek basic details, including brief details of the casualty's illness or injury, type of vessel, next port of call or nearest at which the casualty could be landed, and confirmation of position. If the yacht is mid-ocean, the coastguard will discuss when it is likely to be in range of a helicopter. The coastguard will then put the caller through to a doctor at one of the radio medical advice centres. Medical staff who deal with radio medical advice calls have some familiarisation training so should be aware of the special circumstances and limited facilities likely to be available at sea. Depending on the circumstances and the advice of the doctor, the coastguard may assist in arranging evacuation either by helicopter or lifeboat.

When the caller is put through to a doctor, they will be asked questions to establish the condition of the patient and determine the urgency of the situation. This is known as triage. The caller will be expected to give as much information about the casualty as possible, and should be prepared to write down any instructions they are given.

If using a mobile phone is the only method of communication available, call 999 and ask for the Coastguard.

CASUALTY DETAILS FOR RADIO MEDICAL ADVICE

1	Name	
2	Age	
3	Gender	
4	Can the patient count to ten in one breath?	Yes/No
5	Can you feel a pulse at the wrist?	Yes/No
6	If so, how many beats in one minute?	

7	Responsiveness	Alert	To voice	To pain	No response

8	Skin colour	Pale/cold	Normal	Red/hot

9	Pain (1 = no pain, 10 most severe pain ever)	1	2	3	4	5	6	7	8	9	10

10	Past medical history	
11	Allergies	
12	Medications	
13	Treatment already given	

FIRST AID EQUIPMENT

Many types of first aid kit are available as complete packages commercially or they may be put together with individual items. Any first aid kit needs to be easy to identify, waterproof and readily accessible.

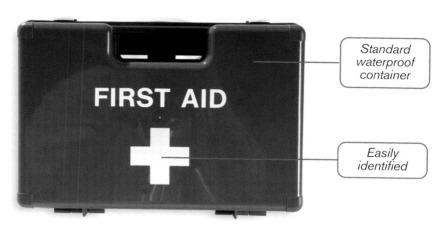

Standard waterproof container

Easily identified

The contents may vary but all will contain the basic dressings. Contents may be supplemented with special dressings. Most will have a manufacturer's expiry date and will be sterile up to that point, as long as the packaging is not damaged.

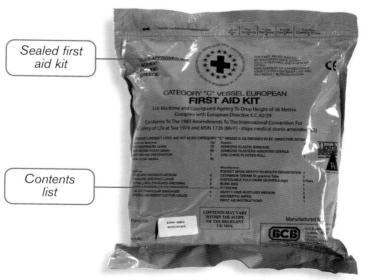

Sealed first aid kit

Contents list

The basic kits should be supplemented accordingly for longer trips and the number of people on board.

BASIC KIT CONTENTS

Sterile wound dressings	Small, medium and large sizes should be in the kit. Small pads also make useful eye pads.
Triangular bandages	A very useful multifunctional dressing. Use for making slings, as a pad, as a bandage to secure dressings or as ties when splinting. They are non fluffy and may be used to cover burns.
Eye pads	An oval shaped dressing pad, which can also be used when small wound dressings are required.
Eye wash solution	Available in small, sterile containers to fit into kits easily, but also available in bottles to store separately. Useful for wound cleaning as well as eye washing. Have a shelf life.
Sterile waterproof adhesive dressings	Different shaped plasters are useful for fingertips or knuckles, for example. Have a variety of types and sizes on board. Hypoallergenic ones are best. Keep all together in a small bag or container inside the main kit to allow quick, easy access.
Sterile gauze swabs	Useful for cleaning wounds and also for providing additional padding over wound dressings.
Disposable non sterile latex-free gloves	Use powder-free gloves, as powdered ones can cause skin irritation. Single use only. Can be purchased in pairs for first aid kits.
Safety pins	Have a selection of sizes for securing bandages and slings. Need to be rustless.
Burn dressings	A number of products are available. They may also contain cooling gel.
Scissors	It is useful to have scissors for cutting dressings and a tough, large pair for cutting off clothing.
Cleaning wipes	These should be individually packed and should not contain alcohol.
Steristrips™	Pre cut adhesive strips used to close small wounds once bleeding has stopped and the wound is clean.
Crêpe bandages	These are elasticated bandages used for supporting sprains and strains. They come in various sizes.

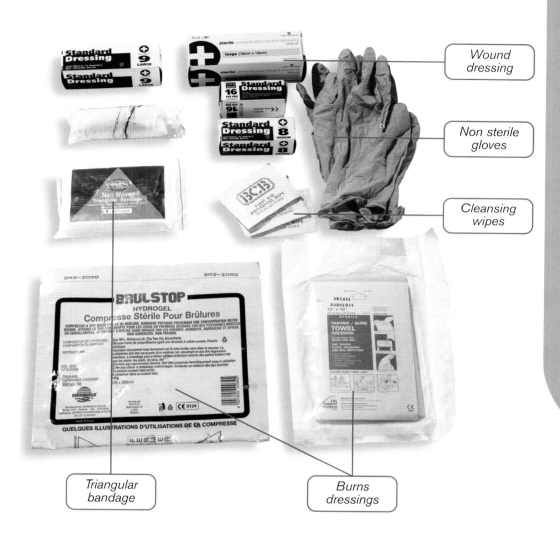

Wound dressing

Non sterile gloves

Cleansing wipes

Triangular bandage

Burns dressings

Other items on board may be used to supplement the basic first aid kit. For example, wet wipes are useful for wound cleaning. Standard wound dressings in first aid kits are quite thin, so if extra padding and absorbency are needed on top of the dressing a sanitary towel may be used. Although not sterile, the individually packed varieties are very clean and have the advantage of absorbency as well as a waterproof backing.

MEDICINES

Medicines should not be kept in the basic first aid kit but in a separate waterproof container. Just as in the home, they should be kept secure if children are on board, to prevent accidental ingestion.

If anyone on board is taking regular medication, it is important to make sure that they have enough supplies with them for the trip.

On short trips, it is sensible to carry some basic items. These would include over the counter products such as paracetamol, ibuprofen and cold remedies. Make sure these are suitable for the age of any children on board. Antiseptic creams, products for burns, seasickness remedies and antihistamines will be useful. Sunscreen is also a sensible item to keep on board.

On longer passages, more medicines will be required in case of emergency, including antibiotics and strong painkillers. These may only be obtained on prescription. Although your GP may be able to advise on what to take and how to obtain it, it is best to go to a company offering a supply service to yachts and merchant vessels. They will be able to provide not only medicines but also any other medical equipment that may be required.

HYGIENE

Preventing cross-infection is part of the role of the first aider. Just as the casualty needs to be protected from infection, so does the first aider.

Contact with blood and body fluids should be avoided where possible by wearing disposable non sterile gloves. These should be worn both when dealing with the injury and when clearing up any spillages and disposing of contaminated materials. Gloves should be kept in the first aid kit. Even though you have worn gloves, you should always wash your hands after contact with the casualty.

As well as wearing gloves to protect yourself, it is sensible to make sure your routine immunisations are up to date.

INDEX

C

D

E

Q

R

sprains 51-3

stable fracture 48

stings 89, 92-93

strains 51-3

stretcher, improvised 106

sunburn 77